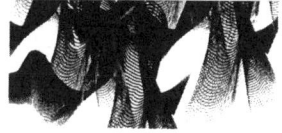

Janice Rider Ellis, F
Professor and Director of N
Shoreline Community Colle
Seattle, Washington

Celia Love Hartley, MN, RN
Professor and Chairperson, Allied Health
Director of Nursing Programs
College of the Desert
Palm Desert, California

Testbank to Accompany

Managing and Coordinating Nursing Care

second edition

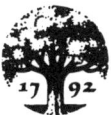

J. B. LIPPINCOTT COMPANY Philadelphia

Sponsoring Editor: Jennifer E. Brogan
Coordinating Editorial Assistant: Danielle J. DiPalma
Ancillary Coordinator: Doris S. Wray
Compositor: Richard G. Hartley
Printer/Binder: George H. Buchanan

Second Edition

6   5   4   3   2   1

0-397-55210-6

Any procedure or practice described in this book should be
applied by the health-care practitioner under appropriate supervision in accordance with professional standards of care used
with regard to the unique circumstances that apply in each
practicce situation. Care has been taken to confirm the accura-
cy of information presented and to describe generally accepted
practices. However, the authors, editors, and publisher cannot
accept any responsibility for errors or omissions or for any consequences from application of the information in this book and
make no warranty express or implied, with respect to the con-
tents of the book.

Every effort has been made to ensure drug selections and
dosages are in accordance with current recommendations and
practice. Because of ongoing research, changes in government
regulations and the constant flow of information on drug thera-
py, reactions and interactions, the reader is cautioned to check
the package insert for each drug for indications, dosages, warn-
ings and precautions, particularly if the drug is new or infe-
quently used.

Preface

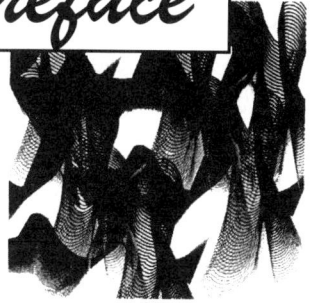

In today's health care system, all registered nurses must be prepared to manage care for groups of patients, manage the health care environment, manage resources for care, supervise the work of unlicensed assistive personnel, and coordinate care with other health care disciplines. In addition, nurses must facilitate the professional development of themselves and others. As the health care environment becomes more complex, consumers increasingly rely on nurses to support them as they move within the sytem.

To move into the role of manager of care, the student needs a foundation of basic information about organization, management skills, and strategies to facilitate working with others. To assist the student in learning these skills, we have developed the text **Managing and Coordinating Nursing Care**. After the publication of the second edition, we received many requests for a testbank that could be used with the book.

The testbank that we have developed in response to the request offers a variety of test formats for each chapter. For each chapter you will find matching questions, short answer questions (which in some instances are based on scenarios), and an assortment of multiple choice questions. The objectives are all keyed to objectives listed at the beginning of each chapter and are intended to provide reference for the instructor. The varying formats allow the instructor to select test questions that best meet the needs of a particular program or style of instruction. Some test questions might best be used in an in-class testing situation. Others are designed so that they could be adapted to a take-home examination. The testbank does not provide answers to the Situations for Critical Thinking posed at the end of each chapter. The open-ended nature of those exercises renders them relatively difficult to cover in a traditional testbank approach.

We hope this testbank will assist and facilitate your instruction. As with the text itself, we welcome your comments and suggestions for improvement.

Janice R. Ellis, PhD, RN
Ceclia Love Hartley, MN, RN

Table of Contents

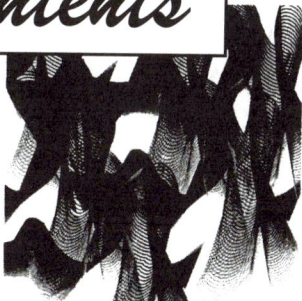

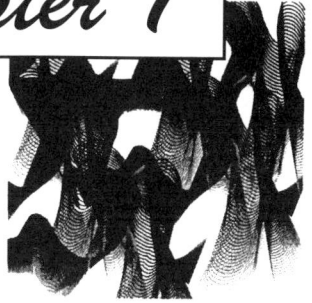

Chapter 1

Becoming a Manager of Patient Care

MATCHING: Match the word in the first column with an explanation in the second column.

Group A

1. achievement-oriented leadership
2. directive leadership
3. participative leadership
4. supportive leadership

___4___ A. The leader focuses on providing encouragement to subordinates.

___1___ B. The leader focuses on identifying and moving toward challenging goals.

___2___ C. The leader focuses on rules and policies.

___3___ D. The leader focuses on joint responsibilities.

(Objective 2)

1

Group B

5. democratic management
6. authoritarian management
7. laissez-faire management
8. multicratic management

_7_ A. Little structure or direction is given to the group.

_8_ B. The leader changes management styles based on the situation.

_6_ C. The leader makes most of the decisions for the group.

_5_ D. Group members are encouraged to participate in decision-making.

Short Answer

Situation A

Sarah Jones, RN, is the evening charge nurse. She always asks the staff to give her input into any decision and often makes the final decision based on the wishes of the majority.

1. Her management style would be termed _____ _____.

   (Objective 2)

2. What is one advantage of the management style described in Situation A?

   (Objective 2)

3. What is one disadvantage of the management style described in Situation A?

   (Objective 2)

Situation B

Michael Schott, RN, serves as the chair of the Nursing Practice Committee for the hospital. The meetings do not have a planned agenda; members of the committee who are interested in a particular topic feel free to suggest it and then to lead the subsequent discussion.

4. This leadership appears to be predominantly what style?

(Objective 2)

5. What is one advantage of the management style described in Situation B?

(Objective 2)

6. What is one disadvantage of the management style described in Situation B?

(Objective 2)

Situation C

Myrtle Myers, RN, is Director of Nursing for a small, privately owned nursing home. She has developed an extensive set of policies and procedures and expects that all staff will adhere to them. Most inservice education is focused on learning these policies and procedures.

7. What is the predominant management style described in Situation C?

(Objective 2)

8. What is one advantage of the management style described in Situation C?

(Objective 2)

9. What is one disadvantage of the management style described in Situation C?

(Objective 2)

10. A colleague states "Good leaders are born, not made." This colleague is supportive of what theory of leadership?

(Objective 1)

11. A nurse reviews her own experience in a variety of situations and says "It is always amazing to me, but when things really get tough or problematic, someone comes forward to help us overcome the problem!" This nurse is giving evidence for what theory of leadership?

(Objective 1)

12. The path-goal theory of leadership focuses on what behavior of the leader?

    (Objective 1)

13. Your new unit manager meets with the staff and as part of her introduction she says "You will find that sometimes I am very task oriented and will push you hard. At other times I will try to pay attention to how you feel and adjust the work demands as best I can. It will depend on the situation." This management style would be termed _____ _____.

    (Objective 3)

14. What is a characteristic of an effective follower?

    (Objective 4)

15. What is one example of nonproductive behavior in a follower?

    (Objective 4)

Multiple Choice

1. According to Fiedler, which of the following has the **most** important influence on the leader's effectiveness?

    A. The size of the organization
    B. The difficulty of the task
    C. Interpersonal relationships between leader and followers
    D. The structure of the organization

    (Objective 1)

2. MBO (management by objectives) is based on

    A.   theory Y management style (human relations management).

    B.   theory X management style (scientific management).

    C.   theory Z management style (Japanese style).

    D.   the premise that the leader must identify the objectives.

(Objective 1)

3. Firm, directive, and limit-setting are terms descriptive of which of the following leadership styles?

    A.   Democratic

    B.   MBWA (management by walking around)

    C.   Authoritarian

    D.   Permissive

(Objective 2)

4. Which of the following leadership styles is considered "people oriented?"

    A.   Laissez-faire

    B.   Authoritarian

    C.   Coercive

    D.   Democratic

(Objective 2)

5. Open, encouraging, cooperation, and recognition are terms descriptive of which of the following leadership styles?

    A.   Democratic

    B.   MBWA

    C.   Authoritarian

    D.   Permissive

(Objective 2)

6. The authoritarian style of leadership would be used in which of the following situations?

   A. A code 99
   B. A workshop planning committee
   C. A research project
   D. A group writing nursing procedures

   (Objective 2)

7. The multicratic manager exhibits which of the following behaviors?

   A. Uses several forms of democratic management technique and tools
   B. Adjusts his or her management style to the situation at hand
   C. Develops the role of the follower to enhance his or her own role
   D. Chooses a management style and sticks to it

   (Objective 3)

8. You are in charge of a group of 16 people (12 nursing assistants and 4 RNs) caring for 88 nursing home residents. Today care must be completed by 1:30 p.m. because of a special event involving most of the employees. Which management style will probably work best in this situation?

   A. Laissez-faire
   B. Authoritarian
   C. Coercive
   D. Democratic

   (Objective 3)

9. Which of the following is NOT a characteristic of an effective leader?

    A. Strong drive for responsibility
    B. Acceptance of interpersonal stress
    C. Intolerance of frustration and delay
    D. Excessive initiative in social situations

(Objective 3)

10. You are in charge of the orientation of a group of nursing assistants who are on the nursing unit for the first time. Which leadership style will probably be most appropriate for you to use?

    A. Democratic
    B. Laissez-faire
    C. Authoritarian
    D. Permissive

(Objective 5)

11. You are a nurse on a busy day surgery unit. You will have a new unit manager beginning Monday. What behavior on your part would best demonstrate that you intend to be an effective "follower"?

    A. Never overstep your role by making suggestions.
    B. Keep quiet about your personal preferences and simply follow the new manager.
    C. Set personal goals that fit into unit goals.
    D. Do not bother the new manager with questions but take them to a trusted coworker.

(Objective 4)

12. Which behavior would be considered acting as an ineffective or poor follower?

    A. Challenge the leader by offering alternative approaches to a problem.

    B. Reevaluate your decision to work in the environment based on newly designed organizational goals.

    C. Let the leader know what you expect of a leader in your environment.

    D. Go along with all decisions of the leader even if you feel they are unwise.

(Objective 4)

13. Which behavior demonstrates a nonproductive management style?

    A. The manager always volunteers to work overtime so the staff does not need to.

    B. The manager tries to help an individual nurse get time off to be with her sick child.

    C. The manager clearly articulates the expectations for staff behavior.

    D. The manager asks staff to vote on a new scheduling system.

(Objective 3)

14. A blizzard has resulted in many staff members being unable to report for work this morning. What management style is most likely to be effective in this situation?

    A. Democratic

    B. Authoritarian

    C. Laissez-faire

    D. It will depend on the preference of the manager.

(Objective 3)

15. Which group is most likely to function effectively with laissez-faire leadership?

    A. A group of clinical nurse specialists newly establishing their roles in a facility
    B. A group of staff that include nursing assistants, unit clerks, licensed practical nurses, and registered nurses
    C. A group of new registered nurses who are being oriented to the facility
    D. A group of patients who have signed up for a class in diabetes management

    (Objective 3)

16. A group leader has announced that all decisions will be reached by consensus. This most closely resembles what leadership style?

    A. Democratic
    B. Authoritarian
    C. Laissez-faire
    D. Multicratic

Answer Key

Matching

Group A	Group B
1. B	5. D
2. C	6. C
3. D	7. A
4. A	8. B

Short Answer

1. democratic
2. (Example) Everyone has a chance for input.
3. (Example) Decision-making may be slower.
4. laissez-faire
5. (Example) Creative input may occur.
6. (Example) The group may fail to focus on goals.
7. authoritarian
8. (Example) Tasks are accomplished.
9. (Example) Group members may feel little personal investment.
10. "great man" theory
11. contingency theory
12. Effort to increase acceptance, satisfaction, and motivation of followers.
13. multicratic
14. (Example) Invests oneself in the organization's goals.
15. (Example) Always portrays the situation as one without solution.

Multiple Choice

1. C	7. B	13. A
2. D	8. B	14. B
3. C	9. C	15. A
4. D	10. C	16. A
5. D	11. C	
6. A	12. D	

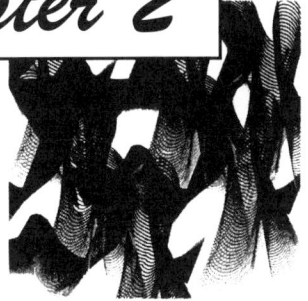

Chapter 2

Understanding Organizational Structure and Function

MATCHING: Match the word in the first column with the phrase or statement in the second.

Group A

1. flat organization
2. tall organization
3. matrix organization
4. informal organization

___ A. Decision-making is reserved to a few people.

___ B. The lines of communication and accountability are complex.

___ C. Authority and accountability are widely dispersed in the organization.

___ D. Is not accountable for outcomes

(Objective 2)

Group B

5. functional assignment

6. primary nursing

7. team nursing

8. case management

___ A. A nurse is assigned to provide all care and assume overall responsibility for a patient.

___ B. A nurse follows the patient's progress throughout the admission, ensuring that care is both timely and appropriate and that outcomes are met.

___ C. A group of nursing staff members care for a group of patients, dividing the work and working together in providing care.

___ D. Each staff member is assigned specific tasks that he or she can do well.

(Objective 4)

Short Answer

1. Why will a nurse find an understanding of organizational structure useful?

(Objective 1)

2. Give an example of a situation in which a nurse might use an understanding of organizational structure.

(Objective 1)

3. Why will a nurse find an understanding of organizational function useful?

(Objective 2)

4. Give an example of situation in which a nurse might use an understanding of organizational function.

    (Objective 2)

5. Draw an organizational chart that represents an organization to which you belong.

    (Objective 3)

6. When you are a nursing student in a clinical setting, to whom are you accountable?

    (Objective 2)

7. If you are the team coordinator on a nursing unit, who would report to you?

    (Objective 2)

8. How might you use an organization's mission statement when seeking employment?

    (Objective 3)

9. Why is an organizational mission statement for a hospital important to clients?

    (Objective 3)

10. What is the purpose of an institutional policy?

    (Objective 4)

11. Why does an institution establish procedures to support practice?

    (Objective 4)

12. Who are members of the informal organization?

    (Objective 5)

13. What purpose does the informal organization serve?

    (Objective 5)

14. What is an organizational climate?

    (Objective 6)

15. How might you affect the organizational climate?

(Objective 6)

16. Give an example of using the knowledge of the informal organization in managing the care of a group of clients.

(Objective 7)

17. Give an example of using the knowledge of lines of authority and accountability in managing the care of a group of clients.

(Objective 7)

18. Give an example of using organizational policies in managing the care of a group of clients.

(Objective 7)

Multiple Choice

1. What is the best definition of an organization?

   A. A legal entity
   B. A business group
   C. A functional group
   D. A formally structured group

   (Objective 1)

2. The organizational structure that is most likely to provide consultant experts to departments or individuals is

   A. tall or centralized.
   B. flat or decentralized.
   C. matrix.
   D. all of the above.

   (Objective 2)

3. In which type of structure are workers more encouraged to participate in decision-making?

    A. Centralized
    B. Decentralized
    C. Matrix
    D. There is no difference.

(Objective 2)

4. The organizational structure in which one individual may have more than one supervisor is

    A. centralized.
    B. decentralized.
    C. matrix.
    D. None is likely to have this situation.

(Objective 2)

5. One of the disadvantages of the tall (centralized) organizational structure is that

    A. it is difficult to determine to whom you report.
    B. there are too many "bosses."
    C. it is difficult to have any degree of expertise.
    D. communication is more difficult because there are so many layers.

(Objective 2)

6. Which one of the following is the best definition of "Span of Control?"

    A. The number of subordinates and tasks for which one person in the organization is responsible
    B. The right one person has to control resources and actions
    C. The responsibility one person has for seeing that the activities are carried out
    D. The way actions occur within an organization

(Objective 2)

7. Which type of organization has few levels?

   A. Centralized
   B. Decentralized
   C. Matrix
   D. None of the above

   (Objective 2)

8. Which type of organization is most likely to have large numbers of formal policies and procedures?

   A. Tall (centralized)
   B. Flat (decentralized)
   C. Matrix
   D. There is no difference.

   (Objective 2)

9. A nurse who is interested in participating in decision-making is most likely to find this opportunity in which type of organization?

   A. Tall
   B. Flat
   C. Matrix
   D. There is no difference.

   (Objective 2)

10. Communication is supported to move through the chain of command in

    A. flat organizations.
    B. tall organizations.
    C. matrix organizations.
    D. all types of organizations.

    (Objective 2)

11. The philosophy of any organization

    A. is needed for legal incorporation.
    B. spells out the broad goals of that organization.
    C. outlines the values and beliefs of members.
    D. identifies the spiritual affiliation of the organization.

(Objective 3)

12. A goal is different from an objective in that it

    A. is more specific.
    B. is measurable.
    C. includes implementation.
    D. is more general.

(Objective 3)

13. Information about who is to make specific decisions for an organization would best be found in

    A. the mission statement.
    B. the policy manual.
    C. the procedure manual.
    D. the job description.

(Objective 4)

14. The need for individuals who value autonomy and increased decision-making is a characteristic of which organization structure?

    A. Tall (centralized)
    B. Flat (decentralized)
    C. Matrix
    D. All of the above

(Objective 4)

15. A characteristic of theory Z management is that

    A.   there are a limited number of decision-makers.
    B.   efficiency is a major emphasis.
    C.   there is concern with feelings and process.
    D.   there is an emphasis on loyalty between employer and employee.

(Objective 4)

16. According to MacGregor's theory Y, workers

    A.   must be rigidly controlled.
    B.   desire security above all else.
    C.   exercise self-control over performance.
    D.   avoid work if possible.

(Objective 4)

17. A basic concept in McGregor's theory X is that people are motivated by

    A.   material gain.
    B.   widely differing things.
    C.   praise.
    D.   accomplishment.

(Objective 4)

18. Policies and procedures

    A.   outline the goals and objectives of any organization.
    B.   provide information about the chain of command.
    C.   are official statements of the organization that guide the behavior of individuals.
    D.   describe the responsibilities of each person within the organization.

(Objective 4)

19. Trading favors is characteristic of the operation of

    A.   the formal organization.
    B.   the informal organization.
    C.   a dysfunctional organization.
    D.   none of these.

(Objective 5)

20. Which of these is a function of the informal organization?

    A.   Establishing lines of authority
    B.   Perpetuating cultural values and norms
    C.   Making decisions within the organization
    D.   Evaluating performance

(Objective 5)

21. In applying Maslow's hierarchy of needs to members of an organization, the informal organization is most likely to meet which needs?

    A.   Belonging/social
    B.   Ego or self-esteem
    C.   Security/safety
    D.   Physiologic

(Objective 5)

22. In an organization in which the housekeeping director and the nursing director are on the same level, both report to a higher level administrator, and both have individual unit managers who report to them, to whom should the staff nurse direct concerns about the adequacy of the cleaning done by an individual housekeeper?

    A.   To the housekeeper individually
    B.   To the nursing unit manager
    C.   To the director of nursing
    D.   To the director of housekeeping

(Objective 7)

23. Given a matrix organizational structure in which each unit manager reports directly to the nursing administrator and works directly with the staff development department, who should do the performance evaluation for the unit manager?

   A. CEO (administrator)
   B. Nursing administrator
   C. Staff development officer
   D. Registered nurse

   (Objective 7)

Answer Key

MATCHING

Group A		Group B	
1. C		5. D	
2. A		6. A	
3. B		7. C	
4. D		8. B	

Short Answer

1. (Example) To work effectively within the organization.
2. (Example) A nurse might use the knowledge of organizational structure to know to whom she is accountable.
3. (Example) To work effectively within the organization.
4. (Example) A nurse might use a knowledge of organizational function to seek a change in nursing procedure.
5. (See chapter for examples of organizational charts.)
6. (Example) Instructor
7. Members of the team
8. (Example) To determine whether your goals are compatible with those of the organization.
9. (Example) It helps the clients understand whether the goals of the organization will meet their needs.
10. To establish who is responsible for decision-making and under what circumstances.
11. To ensure that all employees maintain standards of care.
12. All employees have a role in the informal organization.
13. The informal organization serves many purposes. (Example) It meets the social needs of employees.
14. The prevailing feelings in an organization.
15. (Example) By the way in which you treat others and the way you respond to them.
16. (Example) By understanding who is an informal leader you may be able to support that person in leading toward excellence.
17. (Example) The nurse might seek the assistance of a supervisor to change a policy to meet the needs of the

particular type of patient for whom the nurse is responsible.

18. (Example) The nurse working with a group of cognitively impaired clients might use the policy for who gives consent when the client is not competent to plan for including family in care.

Multiple Choice

1. D	9. B	17. A
2. C	10. D	18. C
3. B	11. C	19. B
4. C	12. D	20. B
5. D	13. B	21. A
6. A	14. B	22. B
7. B	15. D	23. B
8. A	16. C	

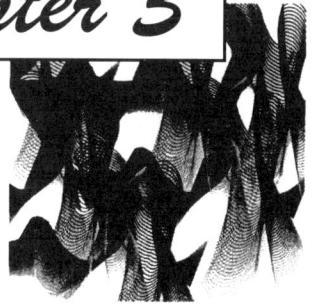

Chapter 3

Managing Resources

MATCHING: Match the word in the first column with an explanation in the second column.

Group A

1. Social Security Act of 1965
2. Tax Equity and Fiscal Responsibility Act
3. Social Security Amendments of 1985
4. health insurance companies
5. Managed Competition Act of 1992

___ A. Placed limitations on payments

___ B. A third-party payer

___ C. DRGs

___ D. Discounted group benefits

___ E. Medicare

Group B

6. control procedures

7. variance

8. cost containment

9. nonsalary cost of care

10 cost awareness

____ A. Includes reduction of waste of limited resources and time

____ B. Buying and distributing supplies, for example

____ C. Used to monitor expenses

____ D. Requires that you understand both personnel and supply costs

____ E. The difference between the expected and the actual

(Objectives 1, 3, and 5)

Short Answer

1. The Medicare program was introduced under the Social Security Act of 1965 to _____.

   (Objective 1)

2. The introduction of diagnostic-related groups in the Social Security Amendments of 1985 brought with it the concept of _____.

   (Objective 1)

3. The largest number of health care dollars is invested by

   _____.

   (Objective 1)

4. Three reasons health care costs have escalated in recent years are _____, _____, and

   _____.

   (Objective 2)

5. Completion of preliminary budgets, budget hearings, completion of a final budget, and presentation of the budget to a final authority are all steps in _____.
   (Objective 3)

6. The use of a systematic approach to the evaluation of products used by an organization is known as

   _____.
   (Objective 3)

7. Capital budget expenditures include _____

   _____.
   (Objective 4)

8. The operating budget is concerned with items that cannot

   _____.
   (Objective 4)

9. Fifty to 60% of a total hospital budget may be that of the

   _____.
   (Objective 5)

10. A position that can be equated to 40 hours per week times 52 weeks for a total of 2080 hours per year may be referred to as a _____.
    (Objective 5)

11. Finding the most cost effective means of accomplishing the desired health care outcomes is a part of

    _____.
    (Objective 5)

12. The nurse's role in cost containment involves _____,
    _____, and _____.
    (Objective 6)

13. The art of delegation is an important part of _____
    _____ through managing time wisely.
    (Objective 7)

14. Recognizing problems before they become major is a significant part of _____.

    (Objective 8)

15. Four ways you might contribute to providing more cost effective care include _____,

    _____, _____,

    and _____.

    (Objective 9)

Multiple Choice

1. John Thomsen, age 76, is admitted to the hospital for a hip replacement. Which of the following would you expect to pay a good share of his hospital bill?
   A. His employer
   B. Medicare
   C. His son
   D. A state insurance plan

    (Objective 1)

2. Which of the following did the Managed Competition Act of 1992 encourage?
   A. Outpatient surgery
   B. Prospective payment
   C. Pay-as-you-go policies
   D. Contracting for discounted group benefits

    (Objective 1)

3. Which is the biggest contributor to hospital cost?
   A. Increased length of stay
   B. Cost of equipment and supplies
   C. Amount of nursing time patients receive
   D. Having surgery

    (Objective 2)

4. What is the basic premise underlying all resource management?
   A. Personnel are most effective when used at their highest level of function.
   B. Supplies are a major cost factor for all hospitals.
   C. Expenditures must be kept at a level below or equal to income over time.
   D. The cheapest way of proceeding may not be the least costly in the long term.

   (Objective 3)

5. Which of the following best describes the budget?
   A. A formal plan for managing financial resources
   B. A projection of future expenditures
   C. A statement of past expenditures
   D. A list of current expenditures

   (Objective 3)

6. How frequently are budgets usually planned?
   A. Quarterly
   B. Semiannually
   C. Annually
   D. Biannually

   (Objective 3)

7. Which of the following is usually included in a budget manual?
   A. The institution's total budget
   B. A listing of administrative costs
   C. Departmental budgets only
   D. Definitions of terms and appropriate budget forms and samples

   (Objective 3)

8. Which of the following items would be listed on the capital money budget of a hospital?
   A. Purchasing a new bulletin board for the visitor's lounge
   B. Salary increased for staff
   C. Installing new ceiling tile and wood flooring in the lobby
   D. An increase in gas heating costs

   (Objective 4)

9. Because of a new contract, you must budget for an increase in nurses' salaries. Under which budget category would you apply for this increase?
   A. Capital budget
   B. Operating budget
   C. Supply budget
   D. Construction budget

   (Objective 4)

10. What is the overall purpose of a budget?
    A. To plan and manage programs and control spending
    B. To identify areas in which excesses are occurring
    C. To save money for the company
    D. To plan for capital expenditures

    (Objectives 3 and 4)

11. In which part of the budget would one find major renovations?
    A. Operating budget
    B. Capital budget
    C. Administrative budget
    D. Equipment budget

    (Objective 4)

12. For what percent of the total hospital budget is nursing often accountable?
    A. 20—25%
    B. 40—45%
    C. 50—60%
    D. 75—80%

(Objective 5)

13. Which of the following greatly influences the patient care hours needed on a unit?
    A. Patient acuity
    B. The ratio of nursing students to staff
    C. Whether nurses have master's degrees
    D. The budgeting process the hospital uses

(Objective 5)

14. What is the process used to monitor expenses called?
    A. Control process
    B. Cost containment
    C. Value analysis
    D. Decision tree

(Objective 6)

15. Which of the following provides the greatest opportunity for cost containment in a nursing department's expenses?
    A. Equipment
    B. Supplies
    C. Environmental assessment
    D. Salaries

(Objective 7)

16. How are vacations, sick leaves, holidays, and staff development days calculated?
    A. As patient care hours
    B. As nonproductive time
    C. As distributive time
    D. As exempt hours

(Objective 7)

17. Of the following, which is the best way in which a staff nurse might become involved in the budget process?
    A. Providing timely budget requests
    B. Reporting to the supervisor extended lunch breaks taken by fellow workers
    C. Looking for ways to reuse supplies
    D. Seeking short cuts to charting

    (Objective 7)

18. Which of the following is the area on the patient's bill where the cost of nursing care has appeared?
    A. Special nursing services
    B. Patient care maintenance
    C. An integral part of "room and board"
    D. Itemized expenses

    (Objective 7)

19. Which of the following is an example of patient care that is not cost effective?
    A. If it is not completed in less time
    B. If it does not meet established standard
    C. If it is completed by unlicensed personnel
    D. If it is not done by an all registered nurse staff

    (Objective 8)

20. To which of the following is risk management related?
    A. Patient safety
    B. Patient acuity
    C. Patient occupancy rates
    D. Patient classification levels

    (Objective 8)

Answer Key

Matching

Group A
1. E
2. A
3. C
4. B
5. D

Group B
6. C
7. E
8. A
9. B
10. D

Short Answer

1. to people 65 years of age and older and to the disabled
2. prospective reimbursement
3. the federal government
4. the increase in average age of the population; costly new technology; greater administrative costs; increased acuity of patients; newer treatments and expensive drugs; increased litigation (any of these)
5. the budget process
6. value analysis
7. changes in the physical plant
8. be reused and are needed for the daily operation of the institution
9. nursing department
10. FTE (full-time equivalent employee)
11. cost containment
12. managing time; managing supplies; participating in planning
13. cost containment
14. anticipatory management
15. conserving supplies; delegating tasks; giving a full day's work for a full day's pay; maintaining patient safety; becoming involved in the budget process (any of these)

Multiple Choice

1. B	8. C	15. D
2. D	9. B	16. B
3. C	10. A	17. A
4. C	11. B	18. C
5. A	12. C	19. B
6. C	13. A	20. A
7. D	14. A	

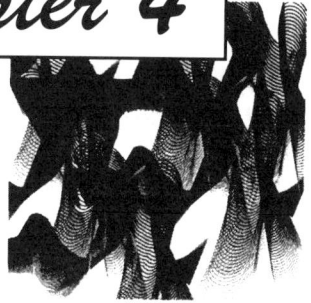

Chapter 4

Understanding and Using Power

MATCHING: Match the word in the first column with the statement in the second column.

Group A

1. personal power
2. position power
3. coercive power
4. information power

___2___ A. The official capacity to exercise control

___3___ B. The ability to require others to act according to your wishes

___4___ C. The ability to accomplish ends based on access to significant data

___1___ D. The ability to act effectively

(Objectives 2 and 5)

Group B

5. expert power
6. connection power
7. referent power
8. reward power

_2_ A. Power arising from collaboration with others

_1_ B. Power arising from the possession of special skills or abilities

_2_ C. Power based in the personal characteristics of an individual

_4_ D. Power based on the ability to provide reinforcement to individuals

(Objective 5)

Short Answer

1. Write your definition of power.

(Objective 1)

2. What nursing position commonly has positional power?

(Objective 2)

3. What are the components of personal power?

(Objective 2)

4. How might legitimate power be used to change a unit policy?

(Objectives 3 and 5)

5. How might reward power be used to encourage student accomplishment in clinical practice?

(Objectives 3 and 5)

6. How might connection power be used by staff nurses to change a policy?

(Objectives 3 and 5)

7. How might you use referent power in your job search?

(Objectives 3 and 5)

8. How might a nurse use expert power?

(Objectives 3 and 5)

9. How might you develop your own personal resources for power?

(Objectives 4 and 6)

10. How might illness affect a client's personal resources for power?

(Objective 4)

11. How might you develop your own expert power?

(Objectives 5 and 6)

12. Describe one action you could take to enhance a client's personal power.

(Objective 7)

13. Describe one action you could take to enhance the power of a nursing assistant with whom you work?

(Objective 7)

14. What type or types of power would be most useful in your obtaining a change in policy regarding visitors in a clinical facility with which you are familiar? For each type identified give one reason it would be useful.

(Objective 8)

15. What adverse responses might occur as a result of your gaining power?

(Objective 9)

Multiple Choice

1. Which type of power is increased by working together with others?

   A. Connection power
   B. Expert power
   C. Legitimate power
   D. Reward power

   (Objective 5)

2. Which is true of power?

   A. All power involves coercion.
   B. A person must have authority to have power.
   C. Power cannot be increased by personal efforts.
   D. Power results in the attainment of goals.

   (Objectives 1 and 3)

3. Which of the following is a true statement about power?

   A. Power usually involves coercion.
   B. You must be aggressive to have power.
   C. Power implies losers as well as winners.
   D. Power includes the ability to achieve intended effects.

   (Objectives 1 and 5)

4. Which one of the following is true of reward power?

   A. It is limited to salary increases.
   B. It can include personal recognition and acknowledgement.
   C. It rests in the hands of a limited number of people.
   D. It is the most difficult type of power to make available.

   (Objective 5)

5. An appropriate use of coercive power might be

    A.   to achieve your goal on a unit.
    B.   to obtain a raise in pay.
    C.   to gain the attention of the management.
    D.   to get a chemically dependent nurse into treatment.

(Objective 5)

6. Which of the following could help you to increase your own power?

    A.   Recognizing and commending others for a job well done
    B.   Increasing your problem-solving and decision-making skills
    C.   Gaining more education
    D.   All of these

(Objectives 4 and 6)

7. Which of the following is another term for authority?

    A.   Referent power
    B.   Reward power
    C.   Coercive power
    D.   Legitimate power

(Objective 5)

8. What is the best description of power?

    A.   Power is the ability to make others do what you want them to.
    B.   Power is a way for a person to be the "winner" in disputes.
    C.   Power provides the ability to produce intended effects.
    D.   Power requires that a person be aggressive.

(Objective 1)

9. Which type of power is increased by attending continuing education events?

   A. Referent power
   B. Expert power
   C. Legitimate power
   D. Reward power

   (Objective 5)

10. The ability to accomplish what you want to accomplish because you are seen as being close to a power person is termed

    A. referent power.
    B. expert power.
    C. coercive power.
    D. reward power

    (Objective 5)

11. What action has the medical profession taken that has undermined nursing power?

    A. Controlled licensure of nurses
    B. Implied to the public that nurses must be dependent
    C. Increased salaries of nonpowerful nurses
    D. Refused to cooperate with nurses

    (Objective 3)

12. A nurse who has the task of deciding how many staff members will be assigned to a unit has what kind of power?

    A. Legitimate
    B. Reward
    C. Coercive
    D. Referent

    (Objective 5)

13. The person who has access to the details of the budget has what type of power?

    A. Connection
    B. Information
    C. Expert
    D. Legitimate

(Objective 5)

14. Which personal base of power is most important to the individual?

    A. See only the good points of yourself
    B. Keep a relaxed attitude
    C. Read extensively
    D. Develop self-esteem

(Objective 6)

15. You have identified that many patients in your long-term care facility are developing catheter-related bladder infections. You would like to change the way catheters are managed. You begin by gathering data on how this problem is managed in other facilities. This is an example of developing what type of power?

    A. Legitimate
    B. Referent
    C. Information
    D. Personal

(Objectives 5 and 6)

16. Which of the following is a common consequence of the use of power?

    A. Increased accountability
    B. Degradation of moral character
    C. Loss of concern for others
    D. Usurpation of authority

(Objective 9)

17. What is the major reason political power is important to nurses?

    A.   To enable nurses to gain greater status
    B.   To prevent the loss of nursing jobs
    C.   To influence decisions about health care funding
    D.   To enhance nursing's image

(Objective 8)

Answer Key

MATCHING

Group A	Group B
1. D	5. B
2. A	6. A
3. B	7. C
4. C	8. D

Short Answer

1. (Example) Power is the ability to accomplish desired ends.

2. (Examples) Chief nursing administrator, director of nursing, unit manager.

3. Personal resources of motivation, self-concept, self-confidence, awareness of personal strengths and abilities, a positive outlook, problem-solving and decision-making ability.

4. (Example) A person with legitimate power (authority) may be able to require that a new policy be developed and actually assign individuals to this task.

5. (Example) A student who does well might be acknowledged by the instructor.

6. (Example) A group of nurses might ask together that a new policy be developed or a current one changed. This would represent more power than would an individual asking independently.

7. (Example) By dressing as a successful and competent person.

8. (Example) If a nurse has previously worked on an oncology unit and is now on a general surgical unit, the nurse might present information from the previous position to demonstrate expertise and then offer a suggestion for care based on this expert knowledge.

9. (Example) Work on my own personal physical health through diet, rest, and exercise.

10. (Example) Illness often creates fatigue that might mean a person would not have the energy to work toward accomplishing a desired goal.
11. (Example) By doing library research on a topic and developing more knowledge than others possess.
12. (Example) Help the client to develop personal expertise in relationship to his or her health status.
13. (Example) Help the nursing assistant to gain information needed to perform the job better.
14. (Example) Expert power. If you were an expert on caring for the specific type of client, others might listen more closely to your proposal than if you were not regarded as an expert.
15. (Example) Others might be distressed that you are taking away some of their power.

Multiple Choice

1. A	7. D	13. B
2. D	8. C	14. D
3. D	9. B	15. C
4. B	10. A	16. A
5. D	11. B	17. C
6. D	12. A	

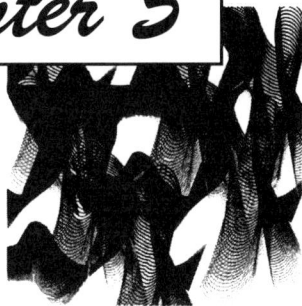

Chapter 5

Using Decision-Making for Quality Care

MATCHING: Match the word in the first column with an explanation in the second column.

Group A

1. realistic
2. feasible
3. ineffective
4. effective
5. systematic

___ A. A decision that it is possible to carry out in light of the resources available

___ B. Decisions that meet or come close to meeting the goals that are established

___ C. A decision that is physically possible or that fits the circumstances or situation

___ D. Characterized by order and direction

___ E. Decisions that do not meet the goals that are established

(Objectives 1 and 4)

Group B

6. autonomy
7. justice
8. beneficence
9. fidelity
10. veracity

_____ A. The commitment to do or bring about good

_____ B. The right of each individual to make one's own decisions

_____ C. The responsibility to carry out the agreements and responsibilities one has undertaken

_____ D. The obligation to tell the truth

_____ E. The obligation to be fair to all people

(Objective 12)

Group C

11 Delphi method
12 brainstorming
13 quality circles
14 task force
15 nominal group technique

_____ A. A group of individuals appointed to work on a specific problem

_____ B. Creating a situation in which selected individuals may think "freely" about a situation and develop creative approaches

_____ C. A group of individuals who volunteer to meet regularly to address common concerns

_____ D. A group of seven to ten individuals who share solutions to a problem, analyze those solutions, and rank them

_____ E. A group of individuals who anonymously share solutions to a problem, analyze those solutions, and rank them

(Objective 9)

Short Answer

1. Decision-making is easier if you _____.

   (Objective 2)

2. The steps in problem-solving and those in the nursing process are _____.

   (Objective 3)

3. The three steps in the decision-making process are

   _____.

   (Objective 3)

4. The step in the decision-making process that is essential to effective planning, action, and evaluation is _____

   _____.

   (Objective 3)

5. Before you can make a decision about a problem, you must _____.

   (Objective 3)

6. Responsibility means that you are _____.

   (Objective 4)

7. Authority infers that you have the _____.

   (Objective 4)

8. We consider a decision to be realistic when it _____.

   (Objective 4)

9. A decision tree is _____.

   (Objective 6)

10. A visual grid that allows us to compare alternative strategies is called a _____.

    (Objective 6)

11. The process of numerical scoring allows us to _____.

    (Objective 7)

12. The task force is frequently used to _____.

(Objective 9)

13. The membership of a quality circle is usually _____
_____.

(Objective 9)

14. When seeking ethical direction in decision-making, two documents that could give assistance are the _____ and _____.

(Objective 12)

15. The process by which individuals are encouraged to assess, explore, and determine their own value system is known as _____.

(Objective 12)

Multiple Choice

1. Which of the following best defines decision-making?

   A. A choice between alternatives
   B. A process by which you solicit input from others
   C. A process, which if logically pursued, always results in positive outcomes
   D. A trial and error process

   (Objective 1)

2. Which of the following is characteristic of persons with good decision-making skills?

   A. They have low intuition levels, so decisions are based on facts.
   B. They use "trial and error" without a logical framework as a guide.
   C. They are able to quickly reduce complex situations into simpler parts.
   D. They are able to quickly make decisions with incomplete or ambiguous data.

   (Objectives 1 and 10)

3. Which of the following is most true of decision-making?

   A. Decision-making is a haphazard process at best and can never be predicted.
   B. Decision-making involves skills that can be learned and improved on.
   C. Good decision-makers are born with skills that facilitate the process.
   D. The best decision-maker is the individual who always involves others in the process.

   (Objective 2)

4. Which of the following best describes the outcome of decision-making?

   A. Approached logically, the results can be predicted.
   B. It is a haphazard process at best.
   C. An authoritarian approach promises the best outcome.
   D. The effectiveness of the approach is totally dependent on the outcome.

   (Objective 2)

5. The steps in the decision-making process are similar to which of the following?

   A. Crisis management
   B. Problem-solving
   C. Fact finding
   D. Triage management

   (Objective 3)

6. Which of the following is a critical element in any decision-making process?

   A. Determining that there really is a problem
   B. Considering every possible solution
   C. Involving others in finding a solution
   D. Setting up a fool-proof method of evaluation

   (Objective 3)

7. Which of the following should you maintain when you have responsibility and accountability for an action?

A. Your sense of power
B. The budget
C. A suitable amount of control over implementation
D. The authority to hire the staff with whom you will be working

(Objective 4)

8. Which of the following best defines a feasible decision?

A. The decision that is the least expensive
B. The decision that creates the least change
C. The decision that is uniformly acceptable
D. The decision that it is possible to carry out in light of the resources

(Objective 4)

9. Which of the following represents an advantage of listing the pros and cons in the decision-making process?

A. The method is simple and direct and can be done quickly.
B. The method involves others in the decision-making process.
C. There is no cost involved in the process.
D. It will always provide for the best solution.

(Objective 5)

10. Which of the following is a disadvantage of listing the pros and cons in the decision-making process?

A. It is expensive and time consuming.
B. It is unreliable.
C. There may be overreliance on both the subjective aspects and the number of the pros and cons.
D. Listing pros and cons will not allow us to really get at the heart of the decision-making process.

(Objective 5)

11. Which of the following is a reason we use a formal approach to decision-making?

    A. It makes the final decision easier and decreases error.
    B. It guarantees the correct answer or decision.
    C. It slows the decision process and results in no need for a decision.
    D. It allows us to visually look at alternatives and compare them.

(Objectives 5, 6, and 7)

12. What is the purpose of a decision tree?

    A. To identify the problem
    B. To ensure the involvement of others in the process
    C. To aid in seeing the critical factors and consequences
    D. To provide a means for evaluating the outcomes

(Objective 6)

13. If you are using a table that includes all pertinent data to be considered to provide a graphic picture to be visually critiqued which of the following are you using?

    A. Matrix or decision grid
    B. Decision tree
    C. Quality square
    D. Table of random numbers

(Objective 6)

Alternative	Cost of Equipment	# of People	Public Relations	Time Needed
#1	$120.00	3	no effect	8 hours
#2	$150.00	2	no effect	4 hours
#3	$280.00	1	no effect	2 hours

14. Which of the following does the above diagram represent?

   A. A decision tree
   B. A decision grid
   C. A decision analysis
   D. A decision algorithm

   (Objective 6)

15. What is one advantage of using a numerical scoring approach to decision-making?

   A. It gives you access to a lot of data.
   B. It is relatively foolproof.
   C. It is relatively simple.
   D. It is not arbitrary or subjective.

   (Objective 7)

16. What is one disadvantage of using a numerical scoring approach to decision-making?

   A. The value attached to the numbers can be arbitrary and subjective.
   B. It is expensive.
   C. It takes too long.
   D. It is an inexact method for approaching decision-making.

   (Objective 7)

17. Which of the following is an important consideration when using group decision-making?

   A. That there is time for group decision-making
   B. That all members of the group can be present for all meetings
   C. That all members of the group have a similar educational background
   D. That the group is compatible

   (Objective 8)

18. Which of the following is a reason we more frequently involve groups in the decision-making process?

    A. Group decision-making is always more effective.
    B. Management approaches today tend to be less authoritarian and involve shared governance.
    C. Management always provides greater support to decisions made by a group.
    D. Group decision-making is less expensive.

(Objective 8)

19. Which of the following involves participative management?

    A. A task force
    B. Decision grids
    C. Listing pros and cons
    D. Numerical scoring

(Objectives 8 and 9)

20. How does a task force differ from a quality circle?

    A. A task force is composed of top management people only.
    B. A task force is randomly selected.
    C. A task force works in anonymity.
    D. A task force adjourns after completion of the task.

(Objective 9)

21. As the charge nurse, if you wanted to involve the staff in helping to plan for dinner rotations you might consider using which one of the following?

    A. The Delphi method
    B. A task force
    C. Majority rule
    D. A department memo

(Objective 9)

22. Which of the following is required if the nurse is to consistently make effective decisions?

  A. A current knowledge base must be maintained.
  B. The team must be composed of persons who are good friends.
  C. There must be uniformity in thinking.
  D. The nurse must have a baccalaureate degree.

  (Objectives 10 and 11)

23. Which of the following is true with regard to ethical decision-making?

  A. Ethical decisions are the responsibility of the physician.
  B. Ethical decisions must always involve an ethics committee.
  C. There are few ethical situations in which nursing is involved.
  D. Ethical decision-making cannot be avoided in nursing.

  (Objective 11)

24. Which of the following best defines the concept of beneficence?

  A. It allows individuals to make their own decisions.
  B. It provides fairness to all.
  C. It is committed to bringing about good.
  D. It ensures that agreements are carried out.

  (Objective 12)

25. Which of the following is the final step in ethical decision-making?

  A. Deciding which decision is best
  B. Taking action and evaluating
  C. Gathering data
  D. Interviewing those involved

  (Objective 12)

Answer Key

MATCHING

Group A	Group B	Group C
1. C	6. B	11. E
2. A	7. E	12. B
3. E	8. A	13. C
4. B	9. C	14. A
5. D	10. D	15. D

Short Answer

1. use a systematic approach
2. quite similar
3. identify and define the area of concern; gather and analyze data; establish goals and desired outcomes
4. establish goals and desired outcomes
5. possess a complete and accurate understanding of the situation
6. accountable and must answer for something
7. power or right to give commands, take action, and make decisions
8. is physically possible or fits the circumstances or situation
9. a graphic tool that allows one to identify the alternative solutions, factors to be considered, and probable outcomes
10. matrix or decision grid
11. weigh the relative merit of alternative strategies
12. address a single problem or concern
13. on a volunteer basis
14. the Code for Nurses; the Patient's Bill of Rights
15. values clarification

Multiple Choice

1. A	10. C	19. A
2. C	11. D	20. D
3. B	12. C	21. B
4. A	13. A	22. A
5. B	14. B	23. D
6. A	15. C	24. C
7. C	16. A	25. B
8. D	17. A	
9. A	18. B	

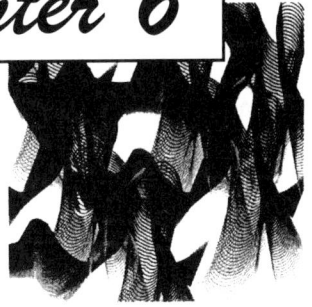

Chapter 6

Organizing Care Effectively

MATCHING: Match the word in the first column with an explanation in the second column.

Group A

1. delegation
2. procrastination
3. work sheet
4. supervision
5. prioritizing

___2___ A. Chronic delay in implementing activities

___3___ B. A "to do" list may be the beginning

___5___ C. Involves putting first things first

___1___ D. Authorizing another person to act in your stead

___4___ E. Involves checking with individuals throughout the day to determine whether they are accomplishing tasks

(Objectives 1 and 2)

Group B

6. effectively	___ A. Steals a great deal of work time
7. efficiently	
8. planning	___ B. Involves taking charge of something
9. controlling	
10. socializing	___ C. Means the situation was made better
	___ D. All endeavors require some of this
	___ E. Means the use of time is maximized

(Objectives 1, 3, and 5)

Short Answer

1. A common expectation of all institutions is that you will be expected to _____.

   (Objective 1)

2. The stress and fast pace of today's world has forced all of us to consider _____.

   (Objective 1)

3. Any endeavor we undertake requires that we spend some time in _____.

   (Objective 2)

4. One of the greatest expenditures of time involves responding to the _____.

   (Objective 2)

5. Meetings should only be called when _____.

   (Objective 2)

6. Keeping your work area free from clutter and distractions helps with _____.

   (Objective 3)

7. A daily work sheet helps to determine what must be done each day and to _____.

    (Objective 3)

8. Techniques to help you with time management include

    _____.

    (Objective 3)

9. When serving as a team leader, one of your first tasks will be _____.

    (Objective 4)

10. A person's success in a leadership role may well relate to the ability to _____.

    (Objectives 4 and 5)

11. It is your responsibility to provide feedback to the persons you are supervising because _____.

    (Objective 5)

12. A key element in supervision is establishing _____

    _____.

    (Objective 5)

13. When you know the capabilities of those with whom you work, you may modify your _____.

    (Objective 5)

14. Often the nurse is responsible for coordinating the efforts of a _____.

    (Objective 6)

15. Time management and organizational skills can also be adapted to assisting a family to _____.

    (Objective 7)

Multiple Choice

1. Which of the following is one PRIMARY advantage of managing our time well?

   A. We will maximize the time and resources we have available.
   B. It will allow us to accomplish a given task faster.
   C. We will be able to do more although it will cost more.
   D. We will accomplish tasks with greater skill.
   (Objective 1)

2. Why are health care facilities primarily interested in staff time management?

   A. It leads to greater staff satisfaction.
   B. The work effectiveness improves.
   C. When time is wasted, money is wasted.
   D. The patients receive more staff time.
   (Objective 1)

3. Which of the following is NOT a time waster?

   A. Phone interruptions
   B. Procrastination
   C. Socializing
   D. Constructing work sheets
   (Objective 3)

4. Which of the following does NOT help change procrastination?

   A. Completing a task a piece at a time
   B. Conserving energy so a task can be completed
   C. Making a commitment to completion of the task
   D. Asking others for more time to do the task
   (Objective 3)

5. Which of the following is true of most procrastinators?

    A. They openly recognize the problem.
    B. They may procrastinate in one situation and not in others.
    C. They are anxious to solve the problem.
    D. They do only priority tasks.

(Objective 3)

6. Before beginning a time management program, a person needs to have which of the following?

    A. An assessment of how time is used
    B. A list of realistic goals
    C. A "to do" list
    D. Knowledge of possible action that can be taken

(Objective 4)

7. You are the charge nurse. Which of the following tasks should you delegate to the LPN (LVN)?

    A. Giving the epidural pain medication
    B. Leading the patient care conference
    C. Counting the linen for inventory
    D. Passing the noon oral medications

(Objective 4)

8. You have just arrived on your nursing unit and discovered you are "in charge." It seems very busy and you are beginning to feel overwhelmed. How will you proceed?

    A. Listen to report, plan your approach, and get to work!
    B. Listen to report, assess the patients, and plan your approach.
    C. Omit report (there isn't time!), get right to assessing your patients.
    D. Delay report and assist the staff currently on duty until things are under control.

(Objective 4)

9. You are the nurse manager. Which of the following should be your priority?

A. A nursing assistant wanting to discuss his vacation time
B. A physician asking that you call him regarding the results of an ordered hematocrit
C. The patient in room 205 who just fell
D. The patient complaining about his lunch and wanting your attention

(Objective 4)

10. You are a senior nursing student. Which of the following tasks might you delegate to the nursing assistant who is helping you?

A. Getting the family a cup of coffee
B. Changing the bed while you ambulate the patient in the hallway
C. Getting the diet tray from the cart while you prepare the patient for a meal
D. All the above

(Objective 4)

11. Which of the following is true of delegation?

A. It is a skill with which one is born.
B. It is a skill that can be learned.
C. It is a skill practiced by registered nurses only.
D. It is a skill that we no longer use.

(Objective 5)

12. Which one of the following is critical when delegating responsibilities?

A. Giving clear instructions
B. Remaining in control
C. Giving everyone a chance to do all activities
D. Keeping accurate notes

(Objective 5)

13. Which one of the following is an important part of the role of the supervisor?

    A. Remaining in control
    B. Monitoring outcomes
    C. Establishing your role as "boss"
    D. Hiring the right people

(Objective 5)

14. What is the purpose of a work sheet?

    A. It must be sent to the nursing office each day.
    B. It keeps track of what you have assigned to whom.
    C. It helps to organize your day and keep track of responsibilities.
    D. It is used only when charting.

(Objective 5)

15. Which of the following is a good reason to have a meeting?

    A. To coordinate action or exchange information
    B. To ensure that everyone is at work
    C. To assert your role as leader
    D. Because people expect frequent meetings

(Objective 6)

16. Which of the following is true of a multidisciplinary team?

    A. The leader must always be a nurse.
    B. The leader is responsible for only the area he or she represents.
    C. The leader may be from another health profession if that is the patient's main reason for health care.
    D. It is much the same as working with a team composed only of nurses.

(Objective 6)

17. Which of the following represents a way in which you can help a family to organize care in the home?

    A. Establishing some strict times for activities
    B. Being certain someone in the family takes the leader role
    C. Helping rearrange the furniture for greater convenience
    D. Setting up some of the same support techniques nurse use in other situations

    (Objective 7)

18. Which of the following is true of home care?

    A. The home health nurse provides care only during brief visits.
    B. The home health nurse is "on call" 24 hours a day.
    C. The home health nurse must visit at least once every 2 days.
    D. The home health nurse keeps a daily journal.

    (Objective 7)

Answer Key

MATCHING

Group A	Group B
1. D	6. C
2. A	7. E
3. B	8. D
4. E	9. B
5. C	10. A

Short Answer

1. organize care effectively and efficiently
2. time management
3. planning
4. requests of others
5. necessary
6. personal organization
7. establish priorities
8. (any of) using work sheets; developing skill in prioritizing tasks; writing things down
9. assessing the group's resources
10. delegate
11. you are accountable for their work
12. effective communications
13. focus in supervision
14. multidisciplinary team
15. organize and provide care in the home

Multiple Choice

1. A	7. D	13. B
2. B	8. B	14. C
3. D	9. C	15. A
4. D	10. D	16. C
5. B	11. B	17. D
6. B	12. A	18. A

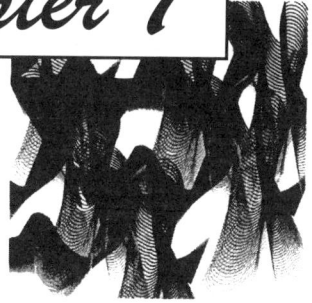

Chapter 7

Providing Feedback and Evaluation

MATCHING: Match the word in the first column with an explanation in the second column.

Group A

1. decode
2. encode
3. narrative technique
4. field review
5. rating scales

___ A. A tool that describes the degree to which a behavior is demonstrated

___ B. Allows the ratings of several supervisors to be compared for the same employee

___ C. Process by which the sender's ideas are converted into the message

___ D. Process by which the receiver interprets the message sent

___ E. The evaluator writes a paragraph or more outlining an employee's strengths and weaknesses.

(Objectives 1, 8, 9, 10, & 12)

Group B

6. positive feedback
7. negative feedback
8. progressive discipline
9. forced choice
10. management by objectives

___ A. Process of evaluating, providing feedback and increasing sanctions on the employee

___ B. Encourages employees' participation in setting their own goals

___ C. Constructive comments

___ D. Communicating unsatisfactory performance

___ E. Choosing from among a group of statements, those that best describe performance

(Objectives 3, 8, 9, & 12)

Short Answer

1. Communication may be defined as _____.

   (Objective 1)

2. The message we send through our physical appearance and movements is considered _____.

   (Objective 2)

3. Some would consider positive feedback a type of _____.

   (Objective 3)

4. Some persons are uncomfortable when they receive any type of feedback, especially _____.

   (Objective 3)

5. We seek and provide feedback to determine that we are_____.

   (Objective 4)

6. The coaching role of the manager is particularly important when it is necessary to _____.

   (Objective 5)

7. A major benefit of performance appraisal to the organization is _____.

   (Objective 6)

8. A major benefit of performance appraisal to the employee is _____.

   (Objective 6)

9. It is critical that an effective performance appraisal be based on _____.

   (Objective 7)

10. In the evaluation process, all individuals have the right to know the _____.

    (Objective 7)

11. Narrative techniques, rating scales, checklists, and management by objectives are all _____.

    (Objective 8)

12. The forced review method is effective in attempting to remove _____.

    (Objective 9)

13. A good feedback interview allows both persons an opportunity to _____.

    (Objective 10)

14. Steps in progressive discipline move from _____
    _____.

    (Objective 12)

15. When involved in a situation requiring progressive discipline, it is important to have _____.

    (Objective 14)

Multiple Choice

1. Which of the following is a characteristic of communication?

   A. It is not influenced by culture.
   B. Emotions have little to do with the manner in which we communicate.
   C. We communicate both verbally and nonverbally.
   D. All communication must be purposeful.
   (Objective 1)

2. In the communication process, decoding involves which of the following?

   A. Creating the idea to be transmitted
   B. Determining the channel by which the message will be sent
   C. Interpreting the message by the receiver
   D. Translating the message into words
   (Objective 2)

3. Which of the following represents the process by which the sender's ideas are converted into the message?

   A. Decoding
   B. Encoding
   C. Validating
   D. Verifying
   (Objective 2)

4. Which of the following is a problem that can occur with any communication process?

    A. The message is usually not complete.
    B. There are many various languages spoken throughout the world.
    C. We clutter our pure language with idioms.
    D. Words can carry different meanings, especially at different stages of development.

(Objective 2)

5. What is one of the major problems related to positive feedback?

    A. It is not given frequently enough.
    B. It is not given with appropriate sincerity.
    C. It is never written down.
    D. It is not used for promotions.

(Objective 3)

6. In what way is feedback critical to evaluation?

    A. It sets the tone of the interview.
    B. It provides information on areas needing modification.
    C. It helps the supervisor and the employee become better acquainted.
    D. It helps to reinforce the job description.

(Objective 4)

7. Which of the following is true of negative feedback?

    A. It should be delayed until the formal evaluation session.
    B. It should be communicated in writing only.
    C. It should be given in private.
    D. It should be provided infrequently.

8. You must speak to an employee for repeatedly using a patronizing form of address for residents, such as "Honey," "Dearie," or "Granny." Where is the best place to talk with this employee?

    A. Wherever she is the next time you hear her address a resident in that way
    B. At the nurses' station
    C. In a private office
    D. In the employee lounge

(Objective 5)

9. Which of the following is a purpose of formal evaluation?

    A. It gives the supervisor something to do.
    B. It orients new employees to the philosophy of the institution.
    C. It keeps a lid on dissension among the "troops."
    D. It targets individuals for promotion.

(Objective 6)

10. Which of the following is true of all performance evaluations?

    A. They should relate to the salary one receives.
    B. They should relate to the job description.
    C. They should relate to the hours one works.
    D. They should relate to whether one works full or part time.

(Objective 7)

11. Which of the following represents a guideline to be used in evaluation?

    A.   The evaluation should always be in writing.
    B.   The evaluation should be conducted at least monthly during the first year of employment.
    C.   The evaluation should be done at the convenience of the supervisor.
    D.   The employee should know who will be doing the evaluation.

(Objective 7)

12. Which of the following is the form of evaluation most often used in letters of recommendation?

    A.   Narrative or essay
    B.   Critical incident
    C.   Rating system
    D.   Checklist

(Objective 8)

13. Which of the following is a disadvantage of the essay technique of appraisal?

    A.   They are difficult to construct.
    B.   They tend to vary greatly in length and content.
    C.   They do not yield depth of information.
    D.   They can have their validity challenged.

(Objective 8)

14. Which type of evaluation tool is probably the most widely used in nursing?

    A.   Narrative or essay
    B.   Checklist
    C.   Rating scale
    D.   Management by objectives

(Objective 8)

15. The medical unit at the university has trained a small group of raters and each rates the employees being evaluated. The ratings are then combined. Why might they be using this approach to evaluation?

    A. To delegate work usually done by the supervisor
    B. To incorporate another aspect of shared governance
    C. To acquaint employees with the evaluation process
    D. To avoid rater bias in the evaluation process

    (Objective 9)

16. Which of the following should be avoided during the performance interview?

    A. Social "chit-chat"
    B. Small talk about work-related situations
    C. The sharing of expectations
    D. The sharing of any negative comments

    (Objective 10)

17. Which of the following is the most appropriate reply when you are complimented for a job well done?

    A. "There was nothing to it."
    B. "Thank you. I appreciate your comment."
    C. "I always try to do my best."
    D. "Ah, gee."

    (Objective 11)

18. If you become upset with information provided to you during a formal feedback session, what should you do?

    A. Tough it out so that your supervisor realizes you "can take the gaff."
    B. Ask to be evaluated by another person.
    C. Request that the interview be terminated and rescheduled at a later date.
    D. Ask to be moved to another unit because this supervisor obviously dislikes you.

    (Objective 11)

19. You receive reports that one of the nursing assistants on your unit is taking supplies to her home. Before speaking with her what would you want to do?

    A. Attempt to observe the behavior.
    B. Collect anecdotal notes from other employees.
    C. Report it to your supervisor.
    D. Search her locker.

    (Objective 12)

20. An employee is consistently late to work. You have documented her lateness over a reasonable period of time. What would you do next?

    A. Ask personnel to deduct the cost of the time missed from her paycheck.
    B. Ignore the lateness because everyone has "emergencies."
    C. Notify the employee that you wish to talk with her.
    D. Suspend the employee.

    (Objective 12)

21. You have observed one of your employees consistently moving from one patient to another without washing his hands. When you talk with the employee about this behavior, which of the following would be the best opening statement?

    A. "You have a bad habit I want to talk to you about."
    B. "I am concerned that you are not taking time to wash your hands between patients."
    C. "I need to put you on formal alert that you are about to receive a reprimand."
    D. "Didn't they teach you about handwashing in the program you attended?"

    (Objectives 12 and 13)

22. After talking with an employee about your concerns for the way she addresses elderly patients, which of the following would be the best concluding statement?

    A. "I am sure I'll never hear you address patients that way again."
    B. "Make sure I never hear you say that again."
    C. "Now that you know what I want from you, do you think you can do that?"
    D. "Please work on changing this behavior and I will talk with you about how it is going next week."

23. In what instance is progressive discipline required?

    A. When you want to set up a coaching situation
    B. When determining that an individual should be transferred to another unit
    C. When an employee's behavior continues to fall below the expected and allowable standard
    D. Before the person completes the first 3 months on your unit

    (Objective 12)

24. Which of the following represents one of the pitfalls that may occur with progressive discipline?

    A. The tendency to be too harsh
    B. The tendency to "overerupt" when "we've had it"
    C. Doing it too early
    D. Overly documenting problem areas

    (Objective 13)

25. An employee who often performed in an unsatisfactory manner when working on your unit asks you to write a recommendation for a job at another hospital. Which of the following should be avoided in your letter?

   A. Writing a glowing evaluation so the employee will get the job
   B. Giving detailed information regarding areas where the employee performed poorly
   C. Using the employee's first name
   D. Indicating that the prospective employer can call you if he has any further questions

(Objective 13)

Answer Key

MATCHING

Group A		Group B	
1.	D	6.	C
2.	C	7.	D
3.	E	8.	A
4.	B	9.	E
5.	A	10.	B

Short Answer

1. the exchange of information
2. nonverbal communication
3. psychological paycheck
4. positive comments
5. sending accurate messages and communicating effectively
6. provide negative feedback
7. improve function of the organization
8. their personal development
9. the job description
10. criteria by which they will be evaluated
11. type of evaluation tools
12. rater bias
13. warm up for the session
14. the least severe to the more critical
15. adequate documentation

Multiple Choice

1.	C	10.	B	19.	A
2.	C	11.	D	20.	C
3.	B	12.	A	21.	B
4.	D	13.	B	22.	D
5.	A	14.	C	23.	C
6.	B	15.	D	24.	B
7.	C	16.	A	25.	A
8.	C	17.	B		
9.	D	18.	C		

Chapter 8

Supporting Competence Through Staff Education

MATCHING: Match the word in the first column with the phrase in the second column.

Group A

1. psychomotor learning
2. affective learning
3. cognitive learning
4. reinforcement
5. learning need

____ A. The learning of attitudes

____ B. Any stimulus that is perceived by the individual as rewarding

____ C. An area in which there is an expectation of knowledge or skill that one does not currently possess

____ D. Learning of skills involving physical tasks

____ E. Pertaining to knowledge of information

(Objectives 2, 5, and 7)

Group B

Match the evaluation strategy with the type of learning for which it is most appropriate.

6. Providing a written test
7. Having a person perform a skill
8. Having a person describe a problem-solving strategy
9. Observing individuals as they interact with patients
10. Orally quizzing an individual

_____ A. cognitive learning
_____ B. affective learning
_____ C. psychomotor learning
_____ D. none of the above

(Objectives 7 and 8)

Short Answer

1. What is competence?

(Objective 1)

2. What ethical statements support the nurse's obligation to maintain competence?

(Objective 1)

3. Why might formal study in addition to practice be necessary for health care team members?

(Objective 2)

4. Identify three avenues for professional development for health care workers.

(Objective 2)

5. What is a major reason that the staff nurse must be responsible for the learning of others on the nursing team?

(Objective 3)

6. Give an example of a way other than teaching that a staff nurse can support the development of another staff member.

(Objective 3)

7. Provide two examples of principles of teaching/learning that apply to staff teaching.

   (Objective 4)

8. Give an example of how you might apply one principle of teaching learning to teaching a nursing assistant.

   (Objectives 4 and 8)

9. What is first essential to assess before beginning to teach any adult?

   (Objectives 5 and 8)

10. What is the first step in planning for staff teaching?

    (Objectives 5 and 8)

11. What are the steps of the teaching process?

    (Objective 5)

12. What is one factor regarding adult education that will affect staff teaching?

    (Objective 6)

13. Where is the center of learning?

    (Objective 6)

14. What are the three major types of learning?

    (Objective 7)

15. What is one problem related to staff education and what is one solution to that problem?

    (Objective 9)

Multiple Choice

1. What is the major ethical reason a nurse must maintain competence?

   A. It is required by law.
   B. The nurse is accountable to the patient for competence.
   C. The ANA has included it in the standards of clinical practice.
   D. The Joint Commission requires it.

   (Objective 1)

2. Marjorie Watson, RN, says that she does not see any need to attend workshops or classes for which she would have to pay. She states that if the hospital does not provide the education then it must not be important in her job. What might you say that would provide an ethical rationale for supporting one's own continuing education?

   A. "You need to go or you might lose your license."
   B. "Your coworkers may think you are behind the times if they learn you never attend anything."
   C. "Nurses have an independent obligation to patients and clients to remain current to provide optimum care."
   D. "You won't get promoted if you do not attend at least some continuing education events."

   (Objective 1)

3. What is the position of the Joint Commission on Accreditation of Healthcare Organizations (JCAHO) regarding staff competence?

   A. The JCAHO does not speak to this issue.
   B. The JCAHO requires that agencies document how they identify and maintain competence of their employees.
   C. The JCAHO requires that all employees have mandatory continuing education.
   D. The JCAHO states that competence is the responsibility of the individual not the agency.

   (Objective 2)

4. If a patient in a hospital or other health care agency receives care that does not reflect the current standard in the community, who might be held responsible?

   A. The individual providing substandard care only
   B. All individuals who cared for the patient and were aware of the substandard care
   C. The agency who employed those who provided substandard care
   D. All of the above

   (Objective 2)

5. What avenue is open to the staff nurse in promoting staff development?

   A. Offering to assist with care so a colleague can attend a class
   B. Planning a staff development program
   C. Providing released time for staff attending continuing education events
   D. Developing a continuing education class

   (Objective 3)

6. As a new graduate, you have identified the need to learn about some of the unit-specific routines. Where is the best place to seek this information?

   A. The staff development department
   B. The unit manager
   C. Policy and procedure books
   D. An experienced staff nurse on the unit

   (Objective 3)

7. The principle that active involvement increases learning is best exemplified by which planning strategy?

   A. Preparing a well-organized lecture
   B. Developing an excellent demonstration of how to do a skill
   C. Preparing interesting and attractive overhead transparencies
   D. Asking staff to develop a schedule for learning activities

   (Objective 4)

8. An example of a reward for learning available for any staff member to use is

   A. a better parking space for those reaching certain continuing education goals.
   B. praise for accomplishment.
   C. an increase in salary for accomplishment.
   D. promotion on the career ladder.

   (Objective 4)

9. Which is a correct assumption pertaining to adult learning according to Knowles?

   A. The center of the learning experience is internal not external.
   B. Adults are less able to learn as they grow older.
   C. Adult learners want someone else to structure and plan the learning.
   D. Adults are more able to deal with situations in which learning does not appear to have immediate relevance.

(Objective 4)

10. Which is a condition related to the learning environment that enhances learning for the adult learner?

   A. A clear line of authority from the teacher is established.
   B. Differences are minimized and all are treated identically.
   C. Guidelines are given as to what is acceptable to discuss.
   D. A feeling of mutual helpfulness is established.

(Objective 4)

11. What is the sequence of steps involved in staff education?

   A. Assessment, planning, implementation, and evaluation
   B. Developing a content outline, planning the approach, and teaching
   C. Identifying the needs of the organization, seeking experts, outlining expectations, providing feedback
   D. Developing lesson plans, carrying out lessons, critiquing lessons

(Objective 5)

12. Sarah Jones, a nursing student, was assigned to care for Wayne Stevens who had surgery yesterday to remove bowel cancer and place a colostomy in the abdomen. She

decides that this morning she will teach him how to irrigate his colostomy. What is the major concern with her approach to this patient?

A. There is no order for irrigation.
B. She has not done any assessment of this individual.
C. This is too soon after surgery to begin any teaching.
D. The patient should have been instructed in colostomy care before the surgery.

(Objective 5)

13. Which factor is most likely to interfere with or support the learning when the staff member is of a different cultural and ethnic background than the nurse?

A. Physical comfort concerns
B. Issues related to mutual trust and respect
C. The freedom of expression that is allowed
D. The helpfulness displayed

(Objective 6)

14. You have a new nursing assistant on your long-term care unit. She is 18 years old and this is her first full-time position since high school graduation. She just finished her nursing assistant training program. What factor will be most prominent in this person's approach to learning?

A. Whether she perceives the learning as meaningful
B. Whether she has resolved her adolescent parental conflicts
C. How successful she was in high school
D. What her major interests are

(Objective 6)

15. You want the staff on the unit to develop a more sensitive approach to persons from different cultures. With which type of learning will you be involved?

    A. Affective
    B. Behavior modification
    C. Cognitive
    D. Psychomotor

    (Objective 7)

16. You will be teaching new skills of managing a patient-controlled analgesia pump to the registered nurses in your long-term care facility. Your planning will be based on the fact that this is what type learning?

    A. Affective
    B. Behavior modification
    C. Cognitive
    D. Psychomotor

    (Objective 7)

17. You intend to work with the staff on their critical thinking skills. This is most accurately categorized as what type of learning?

    A. Affective
    B. Behavior modification
    C. Cognitive
    D. Psychomotor

    (Objective 7)

18. You observe a nursing assistant using poor body mechanics when caring for a patient. Which teaching method would be most effective in changing her behavior?

    A. A formal lecture
    B. An informal demonstration and return demonstration
    C. Having her view a video tape on body mechanics
    D. Having her read a text on body mechanics

    (Objective 8)

19. You will be evaluating the ability of the staff to program the new tube feeding pump. What would be the best method of evaluating their performance?

    A. Providing a written test of the procedures
    B. Discussing the process with each staff member
    C. Observing each staff member program the pump
    D. Asking them to evaluate one another

    (Objective 8)

20. You will be planning a way to assist the nurses in their ability to identify alternatives when faced with patient care problems. Which would be the best way to help them achieve this goal?

    A. Having them read articles about problem-solving
    B. Telling them about successful problem-solving you have done
    C. Providing them with problem situations and have them work in small groups to identify solutions
    D. Providing videos of how to carry out care for specific patient problems

    (Objective 9)

Answer Key

MATCHING

Group A	Group B
1. D	6. A
2. A	7. C
3. E	8. A
4. B	9. B
5. C	10. A

Short Answer

1. (Example) Meeting a standard of skill or ability.
2. (Example) The ANA Code for Nurses.
3. (Example) To obtain basic knowledge or obtain a degree that represents a broad educational background.
4. (Example) Attend conferences, read journals, take courses.
5. (Example) Nurses have an independent obligation to patients for the quality of care provided.
6. (Example) Offer to arrange to substitute for someone so that he or she can attend an education event.
7. (Example) Sequencing of material from known to unknown assists in learning. Active participation of the learner facilitates learning.
8. (Example) Starting with what the nursing assistant knows about bathing patients could be adapted to help the nursing assistant understand how to modify the procedure for a patient with a special skin problem.
9. The current level of knowledge regarding the desired teaching objective.
10. Identifying the desired outcomes or objectives.
11. Assessment, planning, implementation, and evaluation.
12. (Example) The adult learns best what he or she sees as relevant; therefore the teacher must be able to demonstrate the relevance of the learning.
13. (Example) In the individual learner.
14. Affective, cognitive, and psychomotor.

15. (Example) Staff do not attend education events. Provide rewards or reinforcements for those who attend.

Multiple Choice

1. C	8. B	15. A
2. C	9. A	16. D
3. B	10. D	17. C
4. B	11. A	18. B
5. A	12. B	19. C
6. D	13. B	20. C
7. D	14. A	

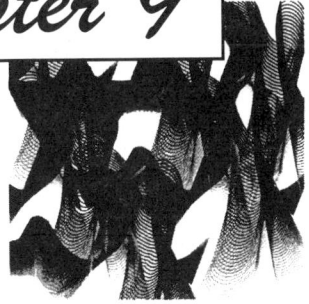

Chapter 9

Motivating Yourself and Others

MATCHING: Match the word in the first column with an explanation in the second column.

Group A

1. affirmation
2. credibility
3. hygiene factors
4. motivators
5. power

___ A. Serve the primary function of preventing job dissatisfaction

___ B. Is a motivator for those who feel a need for control and authority

___ C. Factors that drive behavior

___ D. Positive statements

___ E. The power to inspire the trust and confidence of others

(Objectives 1 and 5)

Group B

6. motives	___ A. Reasons underlying behavior
7. theory X	
8. theory Y	___ B. Can be nurtured by exposing yourself to new ideas
9. enthusiasm	
10 creativity	
	___ C. A mixture of curiosity, confidence, expectation, and optimism
	___ D. Assumes most people would rather be directed
	___ E. Assumes that people naturally enjoy work

(Objective 1, 3, and 5)

Short Answer

1. Motivation might best be described as _____.

   (Objective 1)

2. The factors that drive behavior are considered _____ _____.

   (Objective 1)

3. If you understand what factors influence your motivation you are more apt to _____.

   (Objective 2)

4. Maslow's theory is based on the concept that_____ _____.

   (Objective 3)

5. In Maslow's theory the simplest needs are _____.

   (Objective 3)

6. The theory that we credit to Herzberg may be describe as a _____.

7. McClelland and his associates identified three major motivators, which are _____.
(Objective 3)

8. The theory that suggests that most people find work distasteful and are motivated primarily by physical and security needs is referred to as _____.
(Objective 3)

9. The theory that suggests that most people enjoy work and can be self-directed is referred to as _____.
(Objective 3)

10. Self-motivation, according the Shinn, has two parts. They may be described as _____ and _____.
(Objective 3)

11. A comfort zone may be described as _____.
(Objective 3)

12. Growth means having the courage and confidence to
_____.
(Objective 5)

13. Developing the kinds of habits and skills that will lead you to goal achievement depends in large part on
_____.
(Objective 5)

14. Affirmations help you to _____.
(Objective 5

15. Someone who has taken interest in your development and who will help you work toward achieving your goals is called a _____.
(Objective 6)

16. As a team leader much of your success in directing others will depend on your _____.
(Objective 6)

17. The line between labor and management is becoming

    _____.

    (Objective 6)

18. Credibility might be defined as the ability to

    _____.

    (Objectives 6 and 7)

19. The single most important behavior you can exhibit to
    your staff is _____.

    (Objectives 6 and 7)

20. Positive behaviors that are reinforced by praise

    _____.

    (Objectives 6 and 7)

Multiple Choice

1. Two persons decide to diet and one is successful and one
   is not. To what might we attribute this difference in behavior?

   A.   Their personalities
   B.   The amount of weight each wanted to lose
   C.   Their individual motivation
   D.   Their financial resources

   (Objective 1)

2. Which of the following is a reason you should understand
   theories of motivation?

   A.   To keep up with others
   B.   To be able to enhance your own motivation and
        motivate others
   C.   Your employer will expect this from you
   D.   To move in to a supervisory role

   (Objective 2)

3. In what order are Maslow's hierarchy of needs presented?

   A. From simple to complex
   B. From proximal to distal
   C. From start to finish
   D. From organic to inorganic

   (Objective 3)

4. According to Maslow, which of the following becomes predominate once physiologic needs have been gratified?

   A. Security or safety needs
   B. Need to be loved
   C. Need to be accepted by various groups
   D. Need for self-esteem

   (Objective 3)

5. Who developed the motivation-hygiene theory?

   A. Maslow
   B. McGregor
   C. Herzberg
   D. McClelland

   (Objective 3)

6. Which of the following is most true of McClelland's theory?

   A. It structures needs into a hierarchy.
   B. It deals with affiliation, power, and achievement.
   C. It describes people's attitudes toward work.
   D. It relates people's satisfaction at work with the environment.

   (Objective 3)

7. Which of the following is true of McGregor's theory?

   A. It structures needs into a hierarchy.
   B. It deals with affiliation, power, and achievement.
   C. It describes people's attitudes toward work.
   D. It relates people's satisfaction at work with the environment.

   (Objective 3)

8. Which of the follow is a characteristic of achievement-motivated people?

   A. They consistently earn higher salaries.
   B. They are more often found in management positions.
   C. They are more often among the ranks of the laborers.
   D. They seem more concerned with personal achievement than the rewards these achievements may bring.

9. How might achievement-motivated people be characterized?

   A. They avoid responsibility.
   B. They avoid competitive situations.
   C. They believe they can positively influence outcomes.
   D. They exhibit inconsistent behaviors.

   (Objective 3)

10. Which of the following is a requirement of self-motivation?

   A. You stay within your comfort zone.
   B. You rely heavily on input from others.
   C. You take responsibility for action.
   D. You delegate many responsibilities.

   (Objective 5)

11. Which of the following is important as you strive toward self-motivation?

    A. To weigh your own strengths and weaknesses
    B. To disregard aspects of yourself that are less than positive
    C. To seek assistance from a counselor or friend
    D. To avoid difficult questions regarding yourself

    (Objective 5)

12. Which of the following is a factor that affects work-related motivation?

    A. Attitudes toward authority
    B. Your personality
    C. Your job within the organization
    D. The stable nature of the work ethic

13. Which of the following best describes the concept of shared governance?

    A. It places major responsibility with the supervisor.
    B. It places accountability and authority at the level of the clinical nurse.
    C. It reinforces the leader role of the physician.
    D. It eliminates the nursing assistant from all decision-making.

    (Objective 6)

14. What must first be done to ensure credibility?

    A. Being certain all demands are met
    B. Establishing yourself as someone your subordinates can trust
    C. Securing salary increases for all employees on your unit
    D. Obtaining and posting your job description

15. Which of the following can be identified as a good way to motivate others?

 A. Providing for longer lunch hours
 B. Reducing the time spent in meetings
 C. Providing role model behaviors you want to see
 D. Holding ward conferences on the topic

 (Objective 6)

16. Which of the following is essential in the process of motivating others?

 A. Being certain they understand your role
 B. Being sure that the others want to do the task
 C. Listening to what they have to say
 D. Always delaying your decisions so that they will be more readily accepted

 (Objective 6)

17. Which behavior by the nurse is most likely to increase nursing assistants' motivation to provide high-quality care?

 A. Setting up easy to follow procedures for care
 B. Providing recognition of well-done care
 C. Letting them know whenever care does not meet standards
 D. Avoiding mention of any problems with care

 (Objective 6)

18. Which of the following is true of negative behaviors?

 A. They tend to diminish when rewards are withdrawn.
 B. They are contagious.
 C. They should be reported to the next person in the chain of command.
 D. They should be documented.

 (Objectives 6 and 7)

19. What is one concern expressed regarding constructive criticism?

    A. It may not be understood.
    B. If offered, the subordinate may not "like" you.
    C. It takes a great deal of time to construct.
    D. It does little good because it must be offered in private.

(Objectives 6 and 7)

20. Which of the following is a characteristic of a good working relationship?

    A. It clearly identifies the leaders and the followers.
    B. It ensures that everyone is able to consistently take appropriate breaks.
    C. It results in yearly pay increases.
    D. It is grounded in mutual respect.

Answer Key

Matching

Group A
1. D
2. E
3. A
4. C
5. B

Group B
6. A
7. D
8. E
9. C
10. B

Short Answer

1. the intensity of the will to do, to meet, or to satisfy a need
2. motivators
3. be able to motivate others
4. human needs are ordered in a hierarchy from simple to complex
5. focused on survival
6. motivation-hygiene theory
7. affiliation; power; achievement
8. McGregor's theory X
9. McGregor's theory Y
10. mental; physical
11. all the things with which you are familiar and feel comfortable
12. explore new options
13. your self-esteem
14. (any of) increase your self esteem; project a more confident image; help others see you in a better light
15. mentor
16. ability to motivate those around you
17. more and more blurred
18. inspire the trust and confidence of others
19. a genuine interest in them
20. continue or increase

Multiple Choice

1. C	8. D	15. C
2. B	9. C	16. C
3. A	10. C	17. B
4. A	11. A	18. A
5. C	12. A	19. B
6. B	13. B	20. D
7. C	14. B	

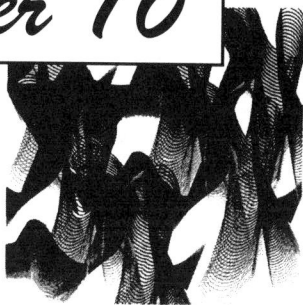

Chapter 10

Evaluating and Improving Patient Care

MATCHING: Match the word in the first column with the phrase in the second column.

Group A

1. continuous quality improvement
2. quality assurance
3. total quality management
4. quality circle

A. Activities used to monitor, evaluate, and control services

B. A process of ongoing analysis and monitoring for the purpose of change

C. A management program to implement quality improvement

D. A team of workers who meet regularly to identify ways of improving outcomes at work

(Objective 7)

Group B

5. goals
6. objectives
7. evaluation standards
8. quality indicator

_____ A. A parameter that might be examined to determine that standards of care are being maintained

_____ B. Specific accomplishment that indicates progress toward a goal

_____ C. Criteria by which accomplishment can be judged

_____ D. Broad statements that indicate the intent of an organization

(Objectives 2, 4, and 5)

Short Answer

1. Name three approaches commonly used for evaluating care.

   (Objective 1)

2. How do goals and objectives differ?

   (Objective 2)

3. What is the difference between a proactive organization and a reactive one?

   (Objective 2)

4. How might personal goals and objectives relate to institutional goals and objectives?

   (Objective 2)

5. What is the focus of quality assurance?

   (Objective 3)

6. Give an example of a common standard used in quality assurance.

   (Objective 4)

7. What is a process standard? Give an example of one.

   (Objective 4)

8. What is an outcome standard? Give an example of one.

   (Objective 4)

9. What is a structural standard? Give an example of one.

   (Objective 4)

10. Where might an organization find standards to use for evaluation?

    (Objective 5)

11. What is the difference between continuous quality improvement and total quality management?

    (Objective 6)

12. What is a key starting point for quality improvement efforts?

    (Objective 6)

13. Describe one key aspect of a quality improvement program.

    (Objective 7)

14. What is the purpose of a quality indicator in a quality improvement program?

    (Objective 7)

15. What is CQI?

    (Objective 6)

16. What is TQM?

    (Objective 6)

Multiple Choice

1. Setting standards for care is a major part of what approach to evaluation?

   A. Quality assurance
   B. Management by objectives
   C. Continuous quality improvement
   D. Scientific management

   (Objective 1)

2. Constant change is characteristic of what approach to evaluation?

   A. Quality assurance
   B. Management by objectives
   C. Continuous quality improvement
   D. Scientific management

   (Objective 1)

3. Establishing general goals for an organization would be important to what approach for evaluation?

   A. Quality assurance
   B. Evaluating relative to objectives
   C. Continuous quality improvement
   D. Scientific management

   (Objective 1)

4. Who would be responsible for determining goals and objectives for the hospital as a whole?

   A. Physicians meeting together
   B. Nursing staff
   C. Board of directors
   D. Community committee

   (Objective 2)

5. Which of the following is the best statement of a personal professional goal?

    A. I will be a better nurse in 1995.
    B. I will complete two courses toward my BSN by the end of 1995.
    C. I will try not to be late so much.
    D. I will attend more continuing education.

(Objective 2)

6. Which should be the more limited, specific statement?

    A. Facility mission statement
    B. Nursing department goal
    C. Nursing unit goal
    D. Quality assurance outcome standard

(Objective 2)

7. According to management by objectives (MBO) principles, who should be involved in formulating objectives?

    A. Top management only
    B. Top and middle management working together
    C. A representative committee
    D. All those who will be working with them

(Objective 2)

8. What is the basic purpose of quality assurance activities?

    A. Maintain a minimal standard of care
    B. Determine whether care is meeting predetermined standards
    C. Identify areas for growth and improvement
    D. Determine whether goals and objectives are being met

(Objective 3)

9. What is expected action when a discrepancy is found between the information collected and the standard?

    A.   The accreditation of the institution will be revoked.
    B.   The state will fine the institution.
    C.   The institution will take corrective action.
    D.   Insurance companies will deny reimbursement.

(Objective 3)

10. "The emergency department shall have a qualified emergency physician present at all times." This is an example of what type of standard?

    A.   Process standard
    B.   Outcome standard
    C.   Structural standard
    D.   All of the above

(Objective 4)

11. "The postoperative infection rate will be no greater than 1% overall." This is an example of what type of standard?

    A.   Process standard
    B.   Outcome standard
    C.   Structural standard
    D.   All of the above

(Objective 4)

12. "An admission nursing assessment will be completed within 6 hours of the patient's admission to an inpatient unit." This is an example of what type of standard?

    A.   Process standard
    B.   Outcome standard
    C.   Structural standard
    D.   All of the above

(Objective 4)

13. "The minimum data set (MDS) will be completed on admission and monthly thereafter for all residents." This is an example of what type of standard?

    A. Process standard
    B. Outcome standard
    C. Structural standard
    D. All of the above

    (Objective 4)

14. Which organization sets general standards for individual nursing performance?

    A. American Nurses Association
    B. Joint Commission for the Accreditation of Healthcare Organizations
    C. Medicare
    D. Insurance companies

    (Objective 5)

15. Which organization sets standards for the function of a nursing department in an acute care hospital?

    A. American Nurses Association
    B. Joint Commission for the Accreditation of Healthcare Organizations
    C. Medicare
    D. Insurance companies

    (Objective 5)

16. In the quality improvement movement where should the power for evaluation be placed?

    A. In the client only
    B. In management only
    C. In employees only
    D. In the client, managment, and employees

    (Objective 6)

17. What is a major focus in all quality improvement activities?

    A. Individual effort is rewarded.
    B. Error is eliminated.
    C. Teamwork is used for problem-solving.
    D. Managers must provide clear directions and guidance in all activities.

(Objective 7)

18. What is the make-up of a "quality circle"?

    A. Managers from different departments meeting together
    B. A manager and his or her immediate subordinates
    C. A group of workers at the same level of the organization
    D. Workers from many different departments

(Objective 7)

19. You have been asked to participate in an audit regarding care of patients with hip fractures. You will be

    A. visiting patient rooms and observing the care given.
    B. meeting with a group of nurses to review care.
    C. planning standards for the care of patients with this diagnosis.
    D. reviewing patient records of individuals who have been treated for a hip fracture.

(Objective 8)

20. The audit in which you are asked to participate will include patients who are still in the hospital. This is what type of audit?

    A. Concurrent
    B. Ex post facto
    C. Prospective
    D. Retrospective

(Objective 8)

Answer Key

Matching

Group A		Group B	
1.	B	5.	D
2.	A	6.	B
3.	C	7.	C
4.	A	8.	A

Short Answer

1. Evaluation by goals and objectives, quality assurance activities, quality improvement activities.
2. Goals are broad and general, whereas objectives are more specific.
3. Proactive means that one identifies potential concerns or problems and takes action to prevent or prepare for them. Reactive means that one waits until a problem occurs and then institutes action.
4. (Example) Personal goals might lead one to choose a specific institution in which to work because its organizational goals matched personal goals.
5. Monitoring, evaluating, and controling services.
6. (Example) The Joint Commission standards for nursing services in a hospital.
7. A process standard identifies the actions that should be taken, their order, and who should take the action. (Example) A standard as to how soon after admission a nursing care plan should have been developed.
8. An outcome standard identifies the desired result of care. (Example) Patients having general abdominal surgery will be discharged without complications by the third postoperative day.
9. A structural standard specifies the building, equipment, and staffing requirements. (Example) Each patient care unit shall have oxygen, suction, and sufficient electrical outlets for the maximum patient care devices expected in the setting.

10. (Examples) The Joint Commission, the American Nurses Association, state practice acts.
11. Continuous quality improvement is a process through which an organization seeks to identify areas for growth or improvement and make changes in those areas. Total quality management is an administrative plan for facilitating continuous quality improvment.
12. A commitment by management to empowering workers.
13. (Example) The use of teams for problem-solving.
14. A quality indicator is information that would indicate that high quality care is being provided.
15. continuous quality improvement
16. total quality management

Multiple Choice

1. A	8. B	15. B
2. C	9. C	16. D
3. B	10. C	17. C
4. C	11. B	18. C
5. B	12. A	19. D
6. D	13. A	20. A
7. D	14. A	

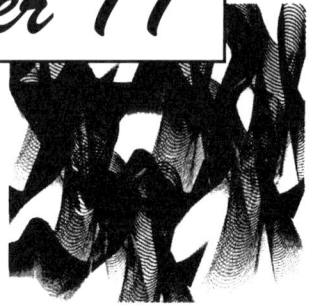

Chapter 11

Managing Change Confidently

MATCHING: Match the word in the first column with an explanation in the second column.

Group A

1. external forces
2. change agent
3. planned change
4. unplanned or reactive change
5. internal forces

___ A. Occurs in response to some event or problem as it arises

___ B. Cause of change originating outside the person or organization

___ C. The person who seeks to cause change

___ D. Cause of change originating within the person or organization

___ E. The deliberate design and implementation of innovation

(Objective 1)

Group B

6. empirical-rational theory
7. co-optation approach
8. power-coercive theory
9. negotiation approach
10. normative-reeducative

___ A. A leader orders change and those with less power comply.

___ B. Change is accepted when it is seen as desirable and is aligned with the interest of those affected.

___ C. Finding areas where both parties can give somewhat and also gain

___ D. Change will occur only after changes have occurred in attitudes, values, skills, and significant relationships.

___ E. Enlisting the opposition onto your theory side by giving them desirable roles in the process

(Objectives 3 and 5)

Short Answer

1. A person who seeks to create or cause change is referred to as a _____.

(Objective 1)

2. Two examples of internal change in nursing that have resulted in an empowered work force and better care are _____ and _____.

(Objectives 1 and 2)

3. If new staffing structures were implemented to create greater employee satisfaction and therefore less staff turnover, this change could be said to come from

_____.

(Objectives 1 and 2)

4. The theory that advocates that a change will be accepted by a person, group, or organization when it is seen as desirable is called the _____ theory.

(Objective 3)

5. The theory of power-coercive change is the basis for _____ and _____.

(Objective 3)

6. The power-coercive strategy for change is best used in situations that _____.

(Objective 3)

7. External and internal forces that push toward change are called the _____.

(Objective 4)

8. Forces that push against change are called _____.

(Objective 4)

9. Lewin's force-field model illustrates the need to look at

_____.

(Objective 4)

10. The first stage in Lewin's sequential model begins with _____ the status quo.

(Objective 5)

11. The last first stage in Lewin's sequential model is called

_____.

(Objective 5)

12. Four factors that may increase the resistance to change could include _____, _____, _____, and _____.

    (Objective 5)

13. One of the key activities in understanding resistance to a specific change is _____.

    (Objective 5)

14. Enlisting key people from the opposition onto your side by giving them desirable roles in the process and thereby ensuring their commitment is called _____.

    (Objective 5)

15. Your first responsibility as a participant in a proposed change is to be sure _____, _____, and _____.

    (Objective 6)

Multiple Choice

1. Which of the following is the term used for the recipients or the target of change?

    A. Change agent
    B. Client system
    C. Champion
    D. Negotiator

    (Objective 1)

2. Which of the following is the term that might also be used for the client system if continuous quality improvement has been adopted?

    A. Change agent
    B. Champion
    C. Negotiator
    D. Stake holder

    (Objective 1)

3. Which of the following best defines external forces?

   A. Changes that originate outside the person or organization
   B. Changes that originate within the person or organization
   C. Changes that have no effect on the person or organization
   D. Changes over which no one in the organization has any control

   (Objective 2)

4. The manager chooses to use an approach to change that involves educating the staff regarding the desirability of the change and how it will affect working conditions. Which theory of change is this manager using?

   A. Empirical-rational
   B. Force-field analysis
   C. Normative-reeducative
   D. Power-coercive

   (Objective 3)

5. Many states have changed their Nurse Practice Act to add sanctions against the chemically dependent nurse. Which theory of change does this exemplify?

   A. Empirical-rational
   B. Force-field analysis
   C. Normative-reeducative
   D. Power-coercive

   (Objective 3)

6. A nurse manager scheduled a series of in-service/work-shop sessions for staff focusing on changing attitudes,

beliefs, and norms. Which approach to change was this manager beginning?

A. Empirical-rational
B. Force-field analysis
C. Normative-reeducative
D. Power-coercive

((Objective 3)

7. Which of the following facilitates the normative-reeducative approach to change?

A. Mutual trust and collaboration
B. Stronger leader participation
C. Selecting a group member to be a leader
D. Inviting consultants to work with the group

(Objective 3)

8. Which process for change involves establishing consequences for noncompliance?

A. Empirical-rational
B. Force-field approach
C. Normative-reeducative
D. Power-coercive

(Objective 3)

9. According to most modern experts, large scale organizational change will not be successful until certain human relations principles are addressed. Which of the following theories of change does this thinking represent?

A. Empirical-rational
B. Force-field approach
C. Normative-reeducative
D. Power-coercive

(Objective 3)

10. On a nursing unit that is changing its pattern of care deliv-
ery, which of the following could be identified as a driving
force?

    A. Increased hours of patient care
    B. Registered nurse's loss of control of patient care
    C. Concern about quality of care
    D. Resistance to training of new staff

(Objective 4)

11. On a nursing unit that is changing its pattern of care deliv-
ery, which of the following could be identified as a
restraining force?

    A. Increased hours of patient care
    B. Decreased cost
    C. Elimination of nonprofessional duties for the
registered nurse
    D. Concern about quality of care

(Objective 4)

12. According to Lewin's theory, at which step in the process
of change is it important to foster new values, attitudes,
and behaviors?

    A. The unfreezing stage
    B. The plan formulation and implementation stage
    C. The refreezing stage
    D. The evaluative stage

(Objective 4)

13. Which of the following must occur to make the need for change greater than the desire to retain the current pattern?

    A. Driving forces are increased and/or restraining forces are decreased.
    B. Driving forces are decreased and restraining forces are increased.
    C. Driving forces are increased and restraining forces are increased.
    D. Nothing is done with either the driving or the restraining forces.

    (Objective 4)

14. Which of the following is an important part of the refreezing stage?

    A. Giving persons opposed to the change an important role to play
    B. Transferring those who still object to the change to another unit
    C. Ignoring all comments about the change that are negative
    D. Giving recognition and reward to those who participated in the change

    (Objective 4)

15. Which step in the change process is often neglected?

    A. Planning
    B. Research
    C. Celebration
    D. Evaluation

    (Objective 5)

16. Which of the following must be done before refining and standardizing any change?

    A. Being certain that all participants have accepted the change

    B. Monitoring the progress and effectiveness of the plan

    C. Developing an alternate plan that can be put into place

    D. Establishing a control group

(Objective 5)

17. Inertia, habit, and comfort with the known may be associated with which of the following?

    A. Unfreezing

    B. Driving forces

    C. Refreezing

    D. Resistance to change

(Objective 5)

18. According to Stoner and Freeman, increasing the driving forces for change may result in which of the following?

    A. Ensuring its success

    B. Leading to hostility and emergence of additional restraining forces

    C. Helping individuals see the need for the change

    D. Increasing the sense of control of the participants

(Objective 5)

19. What is the best thing to do if you have explored the proposed change, its rationale, and its benefits and still find yourself opposed to it?

    A. Express your concerns in a constructive manner.
    B. Seek a transfer to another unit.
    C. Develop and submit a petition signed by yourself and other opposed to the change.
    D. Go along with the change but keep accurate records of the way in which it did not work for future reference.

    (Objectives 5 and 6)

20. Which of the following is your first responsibility as a participant in a proposed change?

    A. Suggest another alternative if you do not agree with the proposed change.
    B. Be sure you understand what the change is.
    C. Determine whether your views are in the majority or minority.
    D. Research the cost of the change.

    (Objectives 5 and 6)

21. Which of the following is true in most real life situations of change?

    A. The empirical-rational theory works best.
    B. The power-coercive theory should be avoided.
    C. The normative-reeducative theory is preferred.
    D. All three of these theories may be operating.

    (Objectives 3 and 6)

Answer Key

Matching

Group A		Group B	
1.	B	6.	B
2.	C	7.	E
3.	E	8.	A
4.	A	9.	C
5.	D	10.	D

Short Answer

1. change agent
2. collective governance; career ladders
3. internal forces
4. empirical-rational
5. regulations; laws
6. bring about a change for the common good
7. driving forces
8. restraining forces
9. multiple factors that can affect the tendency to change
10. unfreezing
11. refreezing
12. (any of) the presentation; timing; pace; weaknesses of the proposal; group's fear; or unwillingness to give up existing benefits
13. listening actively to all objections to the new proposal
14. co-optation
15. you understand what the change is; why it should occur; who will benefit; what is required for success

Multiple Choice

1. B	8. D	15. C
2. D	9. C	16. B
3. A	10. A	17. D
4. A	11. D	18. B
5. D	12. A	19. A
6. C	13. A	20. B
7. A	14. D	21. D

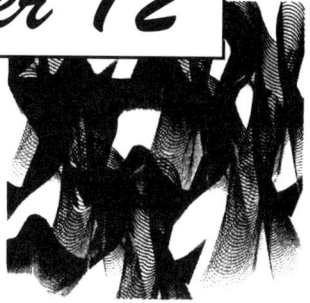

Chapter 12

Meeting and Managing Conflict

MATCHING: Match the word in the first column with an explanation in the second column.

Group A

1. collaborating
2. competing
3. withdrawing
4. smoothing
5. compromising

___5___ A. A give and take approach to conflict

___4___ B. Tries to eliminate anger and expression of difference

___2___ C. Involves working for your particular desired solution exclusively

___1___ D. Individuals work toward common goals

___3___ E. Individual involved chooses not to address the issue at hand

(Objective 6)

Group B

6. consensus
7. lose-lose
8. win-lose
9. negotiate
10. win-win

___9 A. One factor in a situation is balanced against another.

___10 B. Both parties achieve most if not all of their goals or desires.

___7 C. Resolution of the issue is unsatisfactory to both parties.

___6 D. Group members come to agreement.

___8 E. One person dominates the situation and the other individual submits.

(Objectives 6 and 7)

Short Answer

1. In earlier years the traditionalists perceived conflict to be

   _____.

   (Objective 1)

2. Conflict occurs when people with different values, interest, goals, or needs view things _____.

   (Objective 2)

3. When conflict results in lack of recognition of mutual objectives, it would be viewed as _____.

   (Objective 2)

4. The behaviorists of the 1950s began to recognize the

   _____.

   (Objective 2)

5. Today we tend to view conflict as _____.

   (Objective 2)

6. When conflict results in a more equitable allocation of political power or economic resources, it might be viewed as _____.

(Objective 3)

7. When conflict provides the impetus for change, it may be viewed as having _____.

(Objective 3)

8. Role ambiguity occurs when _____.

(Objective 4)

9. Organizations use job descriptions to help minimize conflicts over _____.

(Objective 4)

10. When we debate within ourselves regarding which of two things to do, we are experiencing _____.

(Objective 5)

11. Withdrawing or avoiding a conflict is often seen in people who _____.

(Objective 6)

12. Smoothing or accommodating to conflict is appropriately chosen as an approach when _____.

(Objective 6)

13. Competing or forcing the issue in a conflict involves

_____.

(Objective 6)

14. Compromising or negotiating a conflict situation works because _____.

(Objective 6)

15. The most difficult to achieve but the best approach to conflict is _____.

(Objective 6)

16. The outcomes of conflict resolution can be viewed as cre-
    ating a _____ situation, a _____
    _____, or a _____ situa-
    tion.

    (Objective 7)

17. An important part of resolving any conflict situation
    involves the adroit use of _____.

    (Objective 8)

Multiple Choice

1. When is a conflict said to exist in the interaction between
   two or more parties?

   A. The parties see their goals as incompatible with each
      other.
   B. Neither party is willing to compromise.
   C. Mediators have been called in to deal with the
      situation.
   D. Salaries are being negotiated.

   (Objective 1)

2. Which of the following represents the view of organizational conflict of early writers and theorists?

   A. Conflict is inevitable.
   B. Conflict is to be avoided because it is disruptive.
   C. Conflict can be tolerated because it is energizing.
   D. Conflict can have many positive aspects.

   (Objective 1)

3. Which of the following best represents present-day views of conflict?

    A. Conflict will adversely affect production.
    B. Conflict is to be avoided because it is demoralizing to staff.
    C. Conflict can be an energizing force.
    D. A good manager administers a unit free from conflict.

(Objectives 2 and 3)

4. Which of the following represents one of the positive outcomes of conflict?

    A. Conflict can assist individuals to understand one another's jobs.
    B. Conflict results in greater profits for the organization.
    C. Conflict consistently results in problem resolution.
    D. All feel better because they have had an opportunity to express themselves.

(Objective 3)

5. What is the most frequent cause of group conflict?

    A. Individual frustration and aggression
    B. Unequal sharing of power and rewards
    C. Inequities between classes
    D. Differences in value systems and needs

(Objectives 3 and 4)

6. Which of the following frequently results in conflict within an organization?

    A. Blurring of roles
    B. Job descriptions that are too detailed
    C. Autocratic management
    D. Shared governance

(Objectives 3 and 4)

7. Which of the following does the election of a governor represent?

   A. The exercise of raw authority
   B. Integrative decision-making
   C. Minority rule
   D. Majority rule

   (Objective 6)

8. Which of the following is most apt to be the outcome of negotiation between two "friendly helpers?"

   A. Quick agreement
   B. A stalemate 80% of the time
   C. The need to call in a problem-solver
   D. Resolution of the problem

   (Objective 6)

9. What is the term applied to the situation in which parties work to reach a solution that satisfies the concerns of each?

   A. Collaborating
   B. Compromising
   C. Facilitating
   D. Smoothing

   (Objective 6)

10. How might one classify majority rule?

    A. A win-win situation
    B. A lose-lose situation
    C. A win-lose situation
    D. A situation requiring compromise

    (Objectives 6 and 7)

11. Which personal style is most apt to result in win-win situations?

    A. Tough battler
    B. Compromiser
    C. Problem-solver
    D. Friendly helper

(Objective 7)

12. How might compromise be viewed in a given situation?

    A. A lose-lose situation
    B. A win-win situation
    C. A win-lose situation
    D. Withdrawal

(Objective 7)

13. What is required in the form of conflict resolution that involves consensus?

    A. Reaching agreement among group members
    B. Reaching agreement among the majority of the group
    C. Reaching agreement with 50% of the group plus one
    D. That all members in the group hold similar values

(Objective 7)

14. Which of the following is most apt to result when one of the parties involved in a conflict is intent on meeting his or her own needs?

    A. Lose-lose situation
    B. Win-win situation
    C. Win-lose situation
    D. Withdrawal

(Objective 7)

15. What should occur before one attempts to resolve any type of conflict?

    A. The issues surrounding the conflict should be analyzed.
    B. All parties involved should attend a class on conflict resolution.
    C. A mediator should be "on call."
    D. Attitudes should be adjusted.

(Objective 8)

16. If you are to be responsible for resolving a conflict, what should be your first step?

    A. Examining the issues surrounding the conflict
    B. Talking with all members involved
    C. Seeking the counsel of a mediator
    D. Doing a thorough self-assessment

(Objectives 8 and 10)

17. What is involved in integrative decision-making?

    A. Submission of the issue to a neutral third party
    B. Mental or physical coercion to force compliance
    C. Failure to respond
    D. Joint identification of the needs and values of both parties

(Objective 9)

18. Which of the following is an important ground rule for all conflict resolution?

    A. Everyone talks in turn.
    B. A disinterested third party will be asked to arbitrate.
    C. No one is allowed to belittle another.
    D. All positions should be written out.

(Objectives 8 and 9)

Situation

Two nursing assistants are arguing over whether or not all residents need to be up and dressed for breakfast and one argues that this should be up to the individual. They appeal to the registered nurse to solve the conflict. Questions 19 through 22 refer to this situation.

19. Which of the following best represents the source of the conflict?

    A. A personality conflict
    B. A conflict between staff and management
    C. A conflict based on differences in values
    D. A conflict based on differences in procedures

    (Objective 9)

20. What would be the best approach to managing this conflict?

    A. Attempting to smooth feelings and explain that both ways are OK
    B. Telling them how you want it done
    C. Suggesting that some of the time they do it one way and some of the time they do it the other way
    D. Encouraging them to discuss the reasons they feel the way they do

    (Objective 9)

21. What would be the most significant factor in facilitating the resolution of this conflict?

    A. The group is notified at least one month before the meeting.
    B. The nurse is skillful in negotiating.
    C. There is adequate time for full discussion.
    D. Everyone understands and uses assertive communication skills.

    (Objectives 8 and 9)

22. When evaluating the results of the conflict described above, which of the following is true?

   A. Evaluation should focus primarily on whether or not the conflict itself was resolved.
   B. Evaluation should primarily look at the process to determine whether it was fair to all.
   C. Evaluation should identify permanent policy changes that are needed to prevent this type of conflict.
   D. Evaluation should address both content and process.

   (Objectives 9 and 10)

23. Which of the following is essential to bring about successful conflict resolution?

   A. Assertive communication
   B. Knowledge of techniques of bargaining
   C. A powerful presentation
   D. Clear communication

   (Objective 10)

24. Which of the following should be present if conflict resolution is to be successful?

   A. The parties involved must be willing to negotiate.
   B. A mediator should be hired to work with the group.
   C. People must hold the same values.
   D. People need to understand their role.

   (Objective 10)

25. Which of the following should be considered if the meeting promises to be a volatile one?

   A. Who should be in charge of the meeting?
   B. Limiting the number of persons who will attend
   C. Limiting the damage that can be done
   D. Refusing to deal with inflammatory statements

   (Objective 10)

Answer Key

Matching

Group A	Group B
1. D	6. D
2. C	7. C
3. E	8. E
4. B	9. A
5. A	10. B

Short Answer

1. a disruptive and destructive force within an organization
2. from different perspectives
3. destructive
4. positive aspects of conflict
5. inevitable
6. beneficial
7. positive consequences
8. the expectations of a role are not clear
9. intrapersonal conflict
10. turf; or job responsibilities
11. are made very uncomfortable by conflict situations
12. conflict or anger are disrupting the work setting or interfering with patient care
13. working for your particular desired solution exclusively
14. it minimizes the losses for all persons
15. problem-solving
16. lose-lose; win-lose; win-win
17. interpersonal skills

Multiple Choice

1. A	10. C	19. C
2. B	11. C	20. D
3. C	12. A	21. C
4. A	13. A	22. D
5. D	14. C	23. D
6. A	15. A	24. A
7. D	16. D	25. C
8. B	17. D	
9. A	18. C	

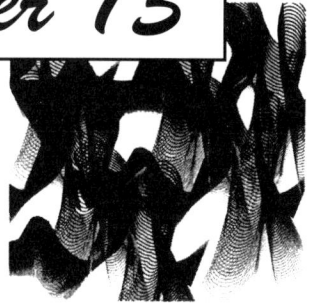

Chapter 13

Becoming an Effective Advocate

MATCHING: Match each term in the first column with a description in the second column.

1. negotiate
2. collaborate
3. empower
4. compromise
5. mediate

_2_ A. Work together with others for a common goal

_1_ B. Interact with others to achieve a change in their contribution or approach to a concern.

_3_ C. Provide another person with the control and authority to act

_4_ D. Find a middle ground between two positions

_5_ E. Interact with two or more individuals or groups to help them achieve a solution to their problem that is satisfactory to all

Short Answer

1. Give two reasons a nurse should assume the role of patient advocate.

   (Objective 3)

2. What is one goal of client advocacy?

   (Objective 4)

3. Describe one strategy for client advocacy.

   (Objective 4)

4. What is a major constraint on the advocacy role?

   (Objective 8)

5. What is a support for the advocacy role?

   (Objective 8)

6. What is one definition of advocacy?

   (Objective 1)

7. List three prerequisites to effective advocacy.

   (Objective 2)

8. List three characteristics that might indicate a client needed an advocate.

   (Objective 5)

9. What is the best strategy for effective advocacy?

   (Objective 6)

10. As a staff nurse, how might you advocate for another health care worker?

    (Objective 7)

Multiple Choice

1. An advocate or ombudsman is one who

   A. protects the rights of all patients within the hospital.
   B. acts as an arbitrator when disputes arise.
   C. acts as a speaker for those who cannot speak for themselves.
   D. supports patient complaints against the institution.

   (Objective 1)

2. Another word that is commonly used for advocation is

   A. helper.
   B. support person.
   C. mediator.
   D. adversary.

   (Objective 1)

3. What is a commonly accepted goal of advocacy?

   A. The client always gets what he or she wants.
   B. The client understands the viewpoint of others in the health care system.
   C. The client no longer has stress within the health care system.
   D. The client copes more effectively with the health care system.

   (Objective 2)

4. Which of the following is essential knowledge for the nurse in becoming a patient advocate?

    A.   The facility's policy on employee handling of patients' rights

    B.   The make-up of the patient population

    C.   The American Hospital Association's Patient Bill of Rights

    D.   The position of the nurses' association in regard to patients' rights.

(Objective 2)

5. Which of the following was an important reason for the development of the advocacy role in health care?

    A.   The expansion of home care where there is minimal supervision

    B.   The increasing use of modern technology in hospitals

    C.   The increasing number of critically ill patients

    D.   The increase in number of residents in nursing homes

(Objective 3)

6. Why should the nurse accept responsibility for the advocacy role?

    A.   The nurse has a unique position from which to gain the trust of the patient.

    B.   This is usually part of the nursing job description.

    C.   No one else in the system understands the patient as well as the nurse.

    D.   Others do not care as much about the patient as does the nurse.

(Objective 3)

7. The patient's physician informs him that he must have chemotherapy or he will die within 2 months. The patient

does not want the treatment. As advocate, you should recognize that the patient

A. has the right to refuse treatment to the extent permitted by law.
B. must recognize the physician's expertise and agree to treatment.
C. has the right to ask for an early death.
D. has an obligation to himself and family to accept the lifesaving treatment.

(Objective 4)

8. Which is the most optimum outcome of advocacy for the client?

A. The client feels someone else cared.
B. The client learns to speak for himself in the health care system.
C. The client expresses trust in health care providers to meet his needs.
D. The client states that his needs have been met.

(Objective 4)

9. Which individual described below most needs an advocate?

A. Mrs. Smith who tells you that she always relies on her husband to decide what is best.
B. Johnny Wilson, age 4, whose mother visits each evening but does not stay the night.
C. Wilmer Stanton, aged 82, who says "Why do people talk over my head as if I were a child?"
D. Mildred Pierce, aged 36, who says "I really wish this surgery were not necessary."

(Objective 5)

10. Advocacy often requires

    A.   aggressiveness and knowledge of policies.
    B.   assertiveness and noncompliance with orders.
    C.   aggressiveness and noncompliance with orders.
    D.   assertiveness and collaboration.

(Objective 6)

11. The hospital patient services representative fulfills which of the following functions?

    A.   Listens to consumer complaints
    B.   Gathers statistical data
    C.   Ensures that a satisfactory resolution will be attempted
    D.   All the above

(Objective 6)

12. A patient shares with you that she thinks her doctor has prescribed the wrong medication and that it is making her "nervous." She is thinking of calling a lawyer. As a staff nurse advocate, you should

    A.   talk privately with the physician.
    B.   mention the conversation to the head nurse.
    C.   encourage the patient to talk with the doctor.
    D.   call the hospital's advocate.

(Objective 6)

13. An elderly woman visits her spouse in the nursing home. She says her doctor told her that if he has another severe heart attack, he'll probably end up a "vegetable." She asks you what this means. Your best reply is

    A.   "You should ask the doctor what he means."
    B.   "He means that he will just lie in bed and not be conscious."
    C.   "I don't know what he means by that."
    D.   "What do you think that means?"

(Objective 6)

14. After talking with you, the above-mentioned woman says she thinks her husband should be "No Code." Your reply is based on the fact that legally, who may make this determination?

 A. The woman
 B. Her husband
 C. The administrator
 D. The doctor

(Objective 6)

15. How might you act most effectively as an advocate in the community to decrease discrimination against persons with AIDS?

 A. Putting brochures on car windshields in the supermarket
 B. Confronting people in social situations about their feelings toward persons with AIDS
 C. Encouraging an organization to which you belong to use AIDS as a program topic
 D. Informing acquaintances about individuals in your community with AIDS

(Objective 6)

16. An effective nurse leader and manager is always an advocate

 A. for the institution in the community.
 B. for each patient in the institution.
 C. for his or her group in the institution.
 D. for his or her group in the community.

(Objective 7)

17. You are the evening charge nurse. A nursing assistant seeks your help in asking the supervisor for a day off for a

special family occasion. What strategy would be the most helpful for this nursing assistant for the long term?

A. Refusing to help to force her to act independently
B. Speaking to the supervisor for her to show her how it is done
C. Encouraging her to replan her family celebration to her usual day off to eliminate the need for special favors
D. Helping her rehearse what she will say to the supervisor when asking for the day off

(Objective 7)

18. What will act as a constraint on the advocacy role of the nurse?

A. The authoritarian atmosphere found in some health care institutions
B. A management system that is decentralized
C. Clients who do not recognize the need for advocacy
D. Lack of support for the role from the professional nursing organizations

(Objective 8)

19. What acts as a support for the advocacy role of the nurse?

A. The legal mandate of patient rights
B. A paternalistic climate in a health care facility
C. Clients who take control
D. A desire to be a "team player"

(Objective 8)

Answer Key

Matching

1. B
2. A
3. C
4. D
5. E

Short Answer

1. (Examples) Nursing values the dignity and autonomy of clients. The ANA Standards support this role for nurses.
2. (Example) Ensure that clients, families, and health professionals are partners, especially when treatment is long, involved, or costly.
3. (Example) Intervene to prevent the need for an advocate through establishing procedures for patients to voice their concerns.
4. (Example) The status of the nurse as an employee.
5. (Example) The patient rights documents.
6. (Example) An advocate defends a cause.
7. (Example) Identification of one's own beliefs and values. Adequate education and experience to be respected. An understanding of the health care system.
8. (Examples) Client has an inadequate knowledge of the health care system. Client is a member of a powerless group (i.e., young child or very old). Client is undecided regarding an ethical dilemma.
9. Preventing the need for advocacy.
10. (Example) Help that colleague to identify ways to speak up for his or her own needs.

Multiple Choice

1. A
2. C
3. D
4. A
5. B
6. A
7. A
8. B
9. C
10. D
11. D
12. C
13. D
14. D
15. C
16. C
17. D
18. A
19. A

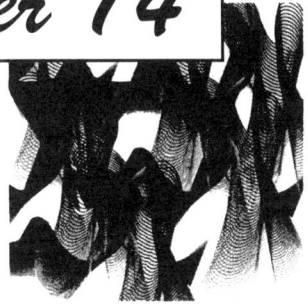

Chapter 14

Understanding and Using Research Findings

MATCHING: Match the word in the first column with a definition in the second column.

Group A

1. control group
2. experimental group
3. subject
4. population
5. sample

___ A. The individuals about whom you wish to seek information

___ B. A representative group of individuals selected for study

___ C. Individuals studied who receive a "treatment"

___ D. Individuals studied who do not receive a "treatment"

___ E. Any individual actually studied

(Objective 1)

Group B

6. validity

7. reliability

8. mortality

9. maturation

10. selection

____ A. The degree to which a given tool actually measures the phenomenon of interest

____ B. Changes in research subjects that are due to outside events that occurred

____ C. The loss of subjects between a first measurement and a second measurement

____ D. The way subjects are chosen that may affect the outcome of the study

____ E. The degree to which a given tool will provide the same measurement on different occasions

(Objective 1)

Short Answer

1. What is the difference between a control group and an experimental group?

(Objective 1)

2. What is the difference between the population and a sample?

(Objective 1)

3. What is the difference between an extraneous variable and an independent variable?

(Objective 1)

4. How does a researcher ensure that consent from a subject meets the standard for informed consent?

(Objective 5)

5. What is the purpose of choosing a random sample for research subjects?

(Objective 1)

6. How are the concepts of probability and significance level related?

(Objective 1)

7. What is the purpose of doing a "triangulation" research study?

(Objective 4)

8. Give an example of a situation that you believe would be appropriate for a quantitative research study.

(Objective 3)

9. Give an example of a situation that you believe would be appropriate for a qualitative research study.

(Objective 3)

10. What was the purpose of the Nuremburg Code?

(Objective 5)

11. List the steps of the research process.

(Objective 2)

12. What is a major advantage of using qualitative research?

(Objective 3)

13. What is a major advantage of using quantitative research?

(Objective 3)

14. What concerns prompted the development of the Nuremberg Code?

(Objective 5)

15. A research report states that the sample used was a convenience sample of those volunteering in a particular clinic. What implication does this have for those interested in applying the results of the study in their own settings?
(Objective 6)

Multiple Choice

1. The first step in designing a research study is

   A. stating the problem.
   B. reviewing the literature.
   C. developing a theoretical framework.
   D. identifying an appropriate population.
   (Objective 2)

2. The purpose of reviewing the literature before beginning a research study is

   A. to determine that the subject has never been studied.
   B. to ensure that you are using the correct approach.
   C. to ascertain what is already known about the problem.
   D. to develop your general knowledge base.
   (Objective 2)

3. What purpose does a theoretical framework serve in a research plan?

   A. It defines the way in which the researcher views nursing.
   B. It ensures that the research will be publishable.
   C. It determines what method will be used for the study.
   D. It supports the conclusions that are drawn.
   (Objective 2)

4. Which is the variable that is manipulated in an experimental study?

    A. Independent variable
    B. Dependent variable
    C. Extraneous variable
    D. Experimental variable

(Objective 2)

5. What is the purpose of a null hypothesis?

    A. It provides statistical clarity.
    B. It means that the researcher does not believe there will be a result.
    C. It specifies the statistical tests that are to be used.
    D. It makes the research more professional.

(Objective 2)

6. What is a characteristic of an experimental research design?

    A. Subjects assigned to groups based on the researchers investigation of their characteristics
    B. Subjects assigned to groups based on their preference
    C. Subjects assigned to groups randomly
    D. Subjects tested both before and after the treatment is applied

(Objective 3)

7. What is a characteristic of a qualitative research design?

    A. The researcher is seeking a contextual understanding of a problem.
    B. The researcher is aiming toward a high degree of research generalizability.
    C. It attempts to provide a measureable approach to subjective data.
    D. It uses specialized statistical tests to determine the significance of the results.

(Objective 3)

8. What is a characteristic of a quasi-experimental research design?

   A. It does not really test anything; it only simulates a test.
   B. It is aimed at describing the phenomenon.
   C. It lacks one or more of the controls of an experimental research design.
   D. It deals with events in the past.

   (Objective 3)

9. A colleague tells you that she does not believe that your institution should change its practices based on a recent research study because she believes the test used lacked reliability. You understand that the colleague believes that

   A. the test does not really measure what it states that it measures.
   B. the test does not produce the same result when repeated.
   C. the subjects were not randomly chosen to take the test.
   D. not enough subjects were studied.

   (Objective 6)

10. Which of the following is considered a quantitative study?

    A. Case history report
    B. Action research strategy
    C. Phenomenology
    D. Ex post facto research

11. You have read a research report and identified that the subjects were all volunteers who responded to a newspaper advertisement. Is there a common problem in this

method of selecting subjects for those wishing to implement the research findings and why?

A. Yes, volunteers are usually unreliable in their responses.
B. Yes, volunteers may not represent the whole population.
C. Yes, volunteers give biased viewpoints.
D. No, volunteers are usually an excellent source of valid and reliable data.

(Objective 6)

12. You have identified that there is no consistent approach to caring for PEG tubes in your long-term care facility. Which of the following people would provide the best consultation regarding setting up a simple research study for your nursing staff?

A. The state surveyor for your facility
B. The administrator for your facility
C. A nursing faculty member who supervises nursing students at your facility
D. The nurse researcher at the tertiary care facility in your state capital

(Objective 6)

13. You have read a research report in which the authors state that although the results are statistically significant they do not appear to be clinically significant. What does this mean to you as a nurse?

    A.   You will probably not see any difference in patients as a result of this treatment.

    B.   Although you will see differences in patients as a result of this treatment, these differences are not related to patient outcomes.

    C.   The study was not reliable enough for the results to be trusted.

    D.   The tool used was not valid for the sample or population being studied.

(Objective 6)

14. A nurse researcher approaches your nursing staff regarding a proposed study that would involve patients on your unit. What are your responsibilities regarding informed consent?

    A.   None, the nurse researcher is responsible for this.

    B.   A research committee at your institution should assume all responsibility for this.

    C.   You should inquire about the plans for consent and not agree to participate if standards have not been met.

    D.   Consent is only a concern if the patients to be part of the study will be subjected to invasive treatments.

(Objective 5)

15. As a beginning staff nurse, what is the role you are most likely to take in nursing research?

    A.   Identifying nursing problems that require research

    B.   Developing a research plan

    C.   Serving as a principal investigator on a research study

    D.   Critiquing the design of proposed research

(Objective 6)

Answer Key

Matching

Group A		Group B	
1.	D	6.	A
2.	C	7.	E
3.	E	8.	C
4.	A	9.	B
5.	B	10.	D

Short Answer

1. A control group does not receive the treatment and is then compared with the experimental group that does receive the treatment.

2. The population is the entire group of people about whom information is desired and the sample is the smaller group that is actually studied.

3. An extraneous variable is one that could affect the independent variable but that is outside of the researcher's control, whereas the independent variable is the one that is manipulated by the researcher for the purposes of the study.

4. By making sure that the subjects receive information in regard to each of the six topics listed in the Nuremburg Code and that they understand their rights as subjects.

5. A random sample ensures that all members of the population had an opportunity to be chosen and therefore differences in the groups are the result of chance.

6. The probability refers to the likelihood that an event will happen. The level of significance is that level of probability that will be accepted by the researcher as representing a true effect and not just the result of chance.

7. Triangulation research provides information from different perspectives, both quantitative and qualitative, and therefore provides a more comprehensive view of the problem.

8. (Example) Any research problem where measurements are needed.
9. (Example) Any research problem where a subjective viewpoint is valuable.
10. To protect the ethical and legal rights of all people who are involved in research.
11. 1) Statement of problem
    2) Review of literature
    3) Development of theoretical framework
    4) Identification of variables
    5) Formation of hypotheses
    6) Selection of research design
    7) Collection of data
    8) Analysis of data
    9) Presentation of findings
    10) Interpretation of findings
12. (Example) It provides a more contextual and comprehensive view of a concern.
13. (Example) It provides more objective and value-free information that may be generalized to a wider population.
14. The experimentation conducted by German researchers on prisoners during World War II.
15. (Example) The results may not apply to other individuals because their response may be biased due to selection.

Multiple Choice

1. A	6. C	11. B
2. C	7. A	12. C
3. A	8. C	13. B
4. A	9. B	14. C
5. A	10. D	15. A